PRAISE FOR
I'VE DECIDED TO LIVE 120 YEARS

*"A delightful guide full of inspiration and information for those
who want to live a full, vibrant, and meaningful life at any age."*

—don Miguel Ruiz
Author of *The Four Agreements*

~

*"This magnificent book ignites the true spirit of what it means to live fully.
But more than that, it provides the precise formula you need to follow if you do indeed
want to live as fully as possible, as healthfully as possible, for as long as possible."*

—Christiane Northrup, MD
Author of *Women's Bodies, Women's Wisdom*

~

*"I have been fortunate to experience firsthand how his visionary view
of the human potential actually translates into reality, and I have incorporated his advice
into my own life. If there is one book you don't want to miss, it is this one."*

—Emeran A. Mayer, MD, PhD
Author of *The Mind-Gut Connection*

~

*"The wisdom here is miles deep yet easily accessible, making it instantly usable.
What you'll read here can change your life for the better immediately,
and you can't ask for more from a book than that."*

—Neale Donald Walsch
Author of the *Conversations with God* series

~

*"Ilchi Lee shines a bright light of ancient and post modern wisdom
on the impact of how each of us defines our life purpose and the pathways
we choose for its fulfillment. His book's genius is not only its . . . principles,
but also how he infuses it with his own good heart."*

—Michael Bernard Beckwith
Author of *Life Visioning*

I've Decided
TO LIVE
120
YEARS

PERSONAL
WORKBOOK

I've Decided

TO LIVE

120

YEARS

PERSONAL
WORKBOOK

ILCHI LEE

BEST
LIFE
MEDIA

459 N. Gilbert Rd, C-210
Gilbert, AZ 85234
www.BestLifeMedia.com
480-926-2480

First paperback edition: June 2018
Library of Congress Control Number: 2018942089
ISBN-13: 978-1-947502-03-1

Cover and interior design by Kiryl Lysenka

CONTENTS

ABOUT THIS PERSONAL WORKBOOK

This workbook is a guide to applying, in a profound, systematic way, the methods of reflection and spiritual practice found in my book I've Decided to Live 120 Years.

This book has been published in English, Korean, and Japanese, and it will soon be available in Chinese, Italian, and other languages. Many readers have reacted passionately to the book. People who once thought of the second half of their lives as a time of decline say that they have corrected their thinking and have been inspired to make it their golden age a time for realizing a life of completion in which they provide for their own health, happiness, and peace. I want to express my heartfelt gratitude for the love and interest of so many readers.

Seeing the reactions of these readers has inspired me to share more with them. So, I began thinking about what they might need and how I could help them. I had the feeling that many readers seriously want to reflect calmly on how they've lived so far and to plan their futures based on their life lessons, as I suggested in my book. I was concerned, though, that—contrary to those desires—they might put off this work, having trouble finding the time in their busy daily lives and not knowing where or how to start.

I decided that people needed a step-by-step guide that anyone could easily follow. I felt a strong sense of responsibility to guide readers, enabling them to actually feel, experience, and apply all the things I'd spoken about in I've Decided to Live 120 Years in their lives. This workbook is an embodiment of that idea and purpose.

Here you'll find supplemental material not covered in *I've Decided to Live 120 Years*, including various questions, instructions, and meditative methods that can lead you through specific, systematic realizations and experiences. You've probably read about three studies needed to grow your soul's energy. The things you've understood and have inspired you through *I've Decided to Live 120 Years* are called the Study of Principles. The Study of Principles is one-third of the course of spiritual work needed to achieve full knowing.

But reading a book once and learning its principles are not enough; two-thirds of the work remains. Knowing is finally complete when it leads to the Study of Practice, which is about directly feeling and experiencing those principles with your body—within all its cells—and to the Study of Living, which is the continuous application of those principles in your life. I hope this workbook guides you into the Study of Practice and the Study of Living, enabling you to engage in a life of completion.

In these pages, you'll find a lot of questions to reflect upon. You don't have to find the answers quickly, as if you were studying for school. I recommend instead that you take time to reflect deeply on the given questions and topics, without rushing. You can close your eyes and meditate or go for a walk and think.

Ponder these questions in your daily life, and you may find that answers suddenly come to mind. There are no right or wrong answers. And no one else can answer for you. Don't look for the answers outside yourself. Instead, continue to seek them in your heart. The answers are within you.

Let me say it up front: this journey is not always easy. However, the process of reflecting on the twists and turns your life has taken so far, of looking into the details of your thoughts, emotions, behavioral patterns, habits, lifestyle, and personal relationships, and of turning the rudder of your life's ship in the direction your true self really wants to go could be a spectacular voyage for you. It might be overwhelming at times, but have patience then. And remember the universal lesson life teaches us all: "No pain, no gain."

The way to get the most out of this workbook is surprisingly simple. Just be honest. You're looking at your life and yourself "just as you are." You don't need to intentionally package, beautify, or justify yourself to look good for someone else or to avoid disappointing yourself. This journey is simply a process for encountering your own truth. Only when you have looked squarely at who you are can intuition and realization finally well up inside you. This is a jewel of wisdom you must dig for within yourself, not a solution someone else brings to you.

Through the diverse methods of introspection presented in this workbook, you will be able to understand and embrace more deeply the being that is you, along with the underlying meaning of your life as you have lived it so far. You can create a more meaningful, fulfilling future based on that acceptance. And you will more clearly identify the life you really want and come up with ideas for making that life a reality.

Most importantly, your life must change substantially. This kind of change begins in your heart. It starts with discovering the nature of your core values, the critical principles that will guide your life. Once you have found those values, you will gain a sure, unshakable center. Then you will be able to center yourself on those values and design your life based on them.

Let me stress this again: all the answers are inside you. So seek the answers within. I hope this workbook will be a wonderful guide and companion as you set out on your journey in search of your true self. Nothing would make me happier than if what I share through this workbook helps even a little to lead you toward a more meaningful, fulfilled, and beautiful life. May you have a meaningful and pleasant journey.

How to Use This Workbook

When you use this workbook, you can go it alone or you can work with others in a book club or other small group.

When you do it alone, take plenty of time and pace yourself. For example, you could go through one chapter a week and set aside more time for the parts you need to ponder longer.

If you want to do it in a small-group setting, bring together people willing to study this workbook with you. You can also recommend it to a book club you already belong to, along with the *I've Decided to Live 120 Years* book.

Since many answers in this workbook must be found alone in deep meditation, I suggest that when you use it with a group, have each person complete the chapter before you come together and then share what each of you wrote and felt. Sharing in this way could be an excellent opportunity to broaden your perspective and understanding of others and to gain vivid life lessons you haven't directly experienced yourself.

All of the materials mentioned in this workbook—the videos, audio, books, and more—can be accessed through Live120YearsBook.com/resources. You'll also find blank pages at the back of this workbook. Use them when you need more space for notes or to record your thoughts. I hope these resources enrich your experience of this essential journey.

I'VE DECIDED TO LIVE 120 YEARS

Read the Introduction and Chapter 1 of *I've Decided to Live 120 Years* before starting this chapter.

We must live as we think, or we shall end up by thinking as we have lived.
—PAUL BOURGET

Check Your Thoughts About Getting Old

How old are you now? _____

Have you ever thought or planned seriously for old age? If not, why not? If you have, write down what you're thinking or planning.

_____

_____

_____

_____

Have you been thinking of old age as a hard, lonely time? Or have you been thinking of it as a time of opportunity and potential to start a new life? Has your thinking about old age been mainly positive or negative?

My guess is that many people will not have thought or planned seriously for their old age. For young people, it may seem like something that is still in the distant future, and it may be that they have too much on their plates to deal with it right now. Even in middle age, old age may seem like some future thing that doesn't feel real because people haven't yet experienced it directly. Until they enter their 60s, people can only have indirect experiences of old age. In other words, all they can do is see the elderly people around them and guess at what old age must be like.

Has anyone close to you—among your family, friends, or neighbors—lived into their old age? Think of people and write down their names and your relationships with them.

I've Decided to Live 120 Years Personal Workbook

Write down in detail what you remember about each of these people: how long they lived, whether they were healthy or suffered from disease, whether they had a happy, meaningful old age.

Did they inspire you to live like them as you got older? Or did you think, "I don't want to live that way"? If so, what was the reason you thought that way?

Have you ever looked at the elderly people around you and tried to guess how many years a person could live an active, healthy life? How many years do you ordinarily think is about right for a life?

Looking at Your Attitude Toward Time

Just a few years ago, I thought that it would be enough to live an active, healthy life until about the age of 80. Then the experience of golfing and talking with 102-year-old Jongjin Lee gave my brain a fresh jolt. It was amazing that such vitality and mental strength could pour from the body of a human over 100 years old.

The first feeling I got from the thought that I could live to be much more than 80 was not anticipation, but the realization that I still wasn't ready. I had thought only that time had been given to me; I hadn't thought that I could extend my time by my will.

What do you usually think about time? Do you tend to passively watch time go by? Or do you actively and intentionally make the most of your time?

Do you believe that people's lifespans are set as if by destiny? Or do you believe that someone can increase or, conversely, decrease their time depending on their individual lifestyle habits and efforts?

Thinking About a 120-Year Life

When I arrived at the thought that I could escape from my passive attitude to actively increase and create my time, I made a choice that would dramatically change my thinking about old age. I decided to live 120 years! What's important is that a clear vision and purpose for what I wanted to achieve through my life came before my choice to live 120 years.

Since choosing to live to 120, I've actively spoken about that choice whenever I've had the opportunity, in private or in public. Most people have been fascinated. Sixty-somethings in particular sit back, relaxed, only to lean forward in their seats and listen carefully when I've talked about this. However, I soon learned that not everyone welcomes my idea. Some have even been antagonistic to my idea of choosing to live to 120. Such people have reacted in one of these three ways:

> ▸ Is that really possible? It's still nothing but a dream.

> ▸ Oh, my God! For me, that would be hell!

> ▸ Just because you made up your mind doesn't mean you're going to live that long, does it? We should just enjoy the years of life given to us before we die.

What about you? Honestly write down whatever thoughts or feelings first came to mind when you saw the title *I've Decided to Live 120 Years* or first encountered talk about a 120-year life.

_____

_____

_____

_____

_____

_____

_____

Our heads are still influenced by ideas from the time when the average lifespan was 60. Without realizing it, we are programmed to think that our 20s and 30s are the time of our youth, and our 40s and 50s are middle age. Thinking of our 60s and above brings to mind infirm bodies, loss, pain, and dependence.

A new method of calculating age was fashionable for a time in Japan, whose people are among the longest lived in the world. According to this method, you multiply your current age by 0.7. Only then, it's claimed, do you get the age you actually feel, physically and mentally, because these days we live much more youthfully than previous generations did.

Using this method of calculation, multiply your age by 0.7. How old does that make you?

_____

_____

Think of that age as the age you actually feel. How does that make you feel?

_____

_____

_____

_____

_____

_____

_____

Calculating age this way, a 50-year-old is 35, a 60-year-old is 42, and a 70-year-old is 49. What about a 120-year-old? 84!

This way of calculating is significant for those of us who think about age from a time when the average lifespan was 60. People generally make the mistake of getting their ideas about old age by looking at the generation that came before them rather than their own generation.

In Korea until just 20 or 30 years ago, when you reached the age of 60 it was normal to invite family and neighbors to a spectacular birthday party. Living to be 60 was no small feat, so everyone would get together to congratulate you on making it to that milestone and to pray that you would have a long life. These days, though, when the average life expectancy is past 80, the age of 60 is still young. Having a big birthday party to celebrate that age has become meaningless and awkward, so the cultural practice mostly faded a long time ago. People these days seem much more youthful at an older age and live longer in good health than people once did.

Try to remember when you were young. Were there people around you then who had passed the age of 60? What were they like? Try to compare them with the people over 60 you see now. What differences do you sense in their health, vitality, and social participation?

_____

_____

_____

_____

_____

_____

_____

_____

_____

_____

You probably read data in the book *I've Decided to Live 120 Years* indicating not only that physiologically a 120-year life is definitely possible, but also that life expectancies are gradually increasing.

- ▸ According to 2015 United Nations data, the number of people over the age of 100 worldwide was then 500,000, a fourfold increase over two decades before, and that growth rate is expected to really pick up speed.

- ▸ The number of Americans over the age of 100 in 2014 had reached 72,000.

- ▸ Average human life expectancy in the United States in 1900 was a mere 47 years, but now it is 79.

- ▸ Average human life expectancy has increased an average of three months per year over the last 200 years.

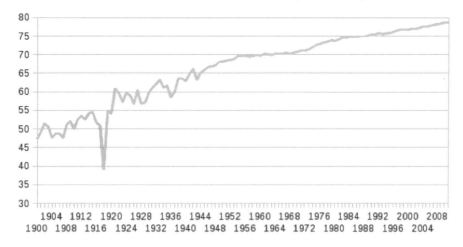

LIFE EXPECTANCY IN THE U.S. (1900–2011)

Source: Centers for Disease Control and Prevention

Thinking About Your Life's Purpose

Before choosing how many years you will live, it's important to have a clear reason and purpose for choosing that number. Having a clear purpose is about giving your life meaning and living it to the fullest. Just extending your life without such a purpose not only has little meaning, but it also could seem greedy.

Reread and get inspiration from the story of Susan Gerace, found on pages 33 and 34 of *I've Decided to Live 120 Years*.

Do you have a purpose that you want to fulfill through your life? If you do, what is it? The following chapters of this workbook will deal with this question in greater depth. For now, just write down whatever thoughts come to mind.

How many years have you chosen to live to fulfill that purpose? This number isn't fixed and can always change in the future, depending on the experiences you have and how your thinking evolves. With a flexible mindset, just write down whatever comes to mind right now.

Choosing a Healthy Lifestyle

Our lives are energy. We are living and breathing now because life energy is operating in our bodies. When our life energy is used up, our lifespans come to an end. It's like a smartphone shutting off if it runs out of battery power. When we reach the bottom line of the minimum life energy needed for our survival, our bodies will stop functioning. Our bodies also break down and stop working when our life energy is blocked and fails to circulate properly, even if a lot remains.

If you understand these principles, you will be able to find hints for a long life here. All we have to do is activate the life energy in our bodies more so it isn't used up or blocked. In other words, we should have lifestyles that stimulate our life energy, like charging a battery, causing our bodies to overflow with vitality.

The power to take the lives we've been given and the authority to decide when they are done ultimately belong to nature, but we can definitely extend the time we have by how we manage our bodies and minds. Those with healthy lifestyles (habits) will have their life energy activated that much more, and those with unhealthy lifestyles will have their life energy activated that much less.

Various studies are demonstrating the link between lifestyle and life extension. The most typical example is exercise. According to a study published in *PLOS Medicine* in 2012, doing the recommended 150 minutes of moderate exercise (or 75 minutes of vigorous exercise) per week yielded approximately 3.4 extra years to one's life. Doing twice the recommended dose meant an additional 4.2 years to one's life. Even doing half the recommended amount made for gains of 1.8 years. According to the researchers' calculations, you gain seven extra minutes of life for every minute of exercise.

Here are some examples of healthy and unhealthy lifestyle.

- **Healthy Lifestyle**

  ▸ Regular exercise
  ▸ Balanced diet
  ▸ Positive thinking

- ▸ Stress management
- ▸ Social interactions
- ▸ No smoking
- ▸ No excessive drinking

- **Unhealthy Lifestyle**
  - ▸ Too little exercise
  - ▸ Unbalanced diet, overeating
  - ▸ Negative thinking
  - ▸ Too much stress
  - ▸ Isolated living
  - ▸ Smoking, excessive drinking

Check your lifestyle. What are your healthy and unhealthy habits? Write them down in the following table, divided into Exercise, Eating Habits, Mindset/Attitude, Personal Relationships, Work/Activity, and Other Areas. (Leave the Eliminate/Reduce and Increase/Create sections empty for now.)

Exercise

Bad Habits	Eliminate/ Reduce	Good Habits	Increase/ Create
Example: I spend a lot of time on the sofa watching TV without moving much.			

Eating Habits

Bad Habits	Eliminate/Reduce	Good Habits	Increase/Create

I've Decided to Live 120 Years Personal Workbook

Mindset/Attitude

Bad Habits	Eliminate/ Reduce	Good Habits	Increase/ Create

Personal Relationships

Bad Habits	Eliminate/ Reduce	Good Habits	Increase/ Create

I've Decided to Live 120 Years Personal Workbook

Work / Activity

Bad Habits	Eliminate/ Reduce	Good Habits	Increase/ Create

Other Areas

Bad Habits	Eliminate/ Reduce	Good Habits	Increase/ Create

I've Decided to Live 120 Years Personal Workbook

Look at the list you've made and mark whether you will eliminate, reduce, or increase each habit. And if there is a new good habit you want to create, add it to the table now.

- **Eliminate:** No longer do what you're doing now.
- **Reduce:** Do less of what you're doing now.
- **Increase:** Do more of what you're doing now.
- **Create:** Add something new that you're not doing now.

Life is a series of choices. Your choices have come together to create who you are now, and they will create who you will be in the future.

This also goes for your lifespan. While walking briskly for 30 minutes, try thinking, "I'm now extending my life by three and a half hours." Try to feel your life energy being activated more fully and your body being charged with more of that energy as you avoid harmful food and eat healthy food, as you think positive thoughts and have joyful conversations with the people around you, and as you get plenty of rest after vigorous activity. Such daily choices will accumulate, extending your life. These are moments when you make a deposit in your longevity account.

That extra time isn't just given to you; you can actively create it through your choices and actions. Isn't that the joy of creation that only we humans can taste and understand?

If, by addressing the questions in this chapter, you have considered your thinking about aging, have chosen the lifespan you want, and have resolved to change your lifestyle actively, then congratulations are in order. If you have felt overwhelmed at all by these life questions, I'd like to encourage you to remember that your journey to a more meaningful and whole life has just begun. As you continue on your journey with this workbook as your guide, your awareness of yourself and what you want will open and deepen, and your ability to choose and take action will strengthen.

Are you encouraged and motivated? Write down what you felt while going through this chapter.

From the list you made of the habits you will change, write down which one you will work on this week.

After working on that habit for a week, write down what changes in the habit you experienced and how they affected your life.

New habits don't form overnight. I hope you will continue to form good habits for longevity and vitality as you continue to repeat these actions for two or three months.

No action, no creation! Change happens when you act.
—ILCHI LEE

CHAPTER 2

WHAT IS HUMANITY'S TRUE PATH?

Read Chapter 2 of *I've Decided to Live 120 Years* before starting this chapter.

If you do not change direction, you may end up where you are heading.
—LAO TZU

Looking at the Paradigm of Success

The life you're living now is the one and only certain opportunity you've been given. No one can definitively prove the existence of past lives or an afterlife. The only certain thing is that *this* life happens only once and cannot be repeated. Shouldn't we live well during the only life we have?

For that, instead of worrying in a fragmentary way over a single event or moment in life, we need to look at the entirety of life from birth to death and really dig into its meaning and essence.

There will be differences from person to person, but let's call the time until the age of 60 the "first half" of our lives and the time after age 60 the "second half." The greatest paradigm permeating the first half of life is "success." Success can be defined as "living well." The problem, though, is when living well and being successful are thought of in a limited way as "winning in competition with others."

What about your own life? What core values have you been pursuing during the first half of your life? In other words, what have you lived passionately for? And how did you work to achieve it?

_____

_____

_____

_____

Do you feel that you've lived a successful life so far, or not? Why do you feel that way?

_____

_____

_____

_____

Think about the goals you've been pursuing, your efforts toward reaching them, and how successful you've been in achieving them at different ages Write your thoughts in the following table.

I've Decided to Live 120 Years Personal Workbook

Age Group	Your Goals	Things You Attempted for Those Goals	Evaluation of Success
Teens			
20s			
30s			
40s			
50s			
After 60s			

In a social system tightly integrated with the paradigm of success, people have no time to consider why they thirst for success or rush into unlimited competition. Caught up in the rat race, they're busy just trying to survive day to day in a social system put together that way.

But let's stop and think for a moment. Why, how, and for how long have we had this obsession with being successful? Is success really the only paradigm available to us?

Look back on your life and consider the idea, "I have to be successful. I have to beat the competition." Who or what formed that idea? You were probably influenced by your parents, family, friends, school, and the media. Write down in detail what stories you've heard and what information you received from others.

Think about the goals you entered in the table for each age grouping. What were your reasons and motives for establishing those goals? Were they chosen by your true self, or were they affected by your parents, other people, or the social system? Consider this question for each age group.

Age Group	Reasons & Motives for Goals	Source of Your Motives
Teens		
20s		
30s		
40s		
50s		
After 60s		

Finding a New Paradigm for the Second Half of Life

In the first half of our lives, we've had the paradigm of "success," which has permeated all of society. So every time the question arises in their minds, "Is this really living well?" people comfort themselves by thinking, "What's the big deal about life, anyway? It's enough to just live the way everybody else does."

We've been busy living day by day as somebody's son or daughter, as someone's mother or father, as someone's partner, or as the title written on our business cards. As our social and family responsibilities decrease in the second half of our lives, though, we encounter a time when our choices can exert more power than the tags that have defined us up to now.

What, then, will you consider your core values, and what purpose and goals will you have? Even if you're too young to think about retirement now, it will definitely be meaningful to reflect on the core values of your life that you would like to have going forward.

In the future or during the second half of your life, do you want to keep going in the same direction you have so far? Or do you want to change things up? What is your reason for feeling that way?

If you want to set a new direction for your life, it's probably because you've discovered that something has been missing. Thinking back on your life, what do you feel has been lacking or unsatisfactory?

What life direction do you want to pursue in the future? What do you want to have as your purpose for the rest of your life?

Whatever you've established as your new purpose, I believe that it probably comes from a desire for greater fulfillment and meaning in the inner quality of your life rather than its external appearance.

All of us probably have in our hearts a desire to grow and develop more today than yesterday, to have the freedom and awareness to care for those around us instead of just ourselves, to proudly and confidently deal with others and ourselves based on a deeper, broader perspective, and to continue loving and creating our lives with greater positivity.

The earnest desire to cultivate ourselves internally, developing greater maturity and fullness—this I express with the word completion. I believe that we all have within us a fundamental desire to make ourselves and our lives fuller and more complete.

Do you have a desire for completion? Are there moments when you feel an earnest desire to cultivate yourself internally, developing greater maturity and fullness? If you do, then write down in detail when you feel that way and how you feel at those times.

The desire for completion is inherent in everyone. According to a book written by Australian palliative care nurse Bronnie Ware, *The Top Five Regrets of the Dying*, these are the most common regrets of people facing death:

1. I should have had the courage to live a life that was true to myself, not the life others expected of me.

2. I shouldn't have worked so much.

3. I should have had the courage to express my feelings.

4. I should have stayed in contact with my friends.

5. I should have made myself happier.

A common feature here is regret over failing to find inner happiness and satisfaction—not regret over failing to find material satisfaction, not "I should have made more money" or "I should have owned more."

The fact that the main standard of measure for evaluating our lives before death is inner satisfaction, not external success, is highly suggestive. Here we find a longing for fulfillment and the completion of ourselves and our lives. People who feel that their lives were full and complete assess their life satisfaction highly, and as a result they feel pride and peace about their lives. But those who feel that something was missing from their lives—that they were not fulfilling—rate their life satisfaction low and have regrets about what they feel was missing.

Everyone has an innate sense for assessing their satisfaction with life—in other words, its level of completion. Completion is something you can fully realize for yourself, without anyone else judging it for you. And it's contradictory for another person to assess this, for only you can know the truth about yourself.

How satisfied are you with your life so far? Draw lines or use color to fill in the portion of the following circle that indicates how much satisfaction you feel.

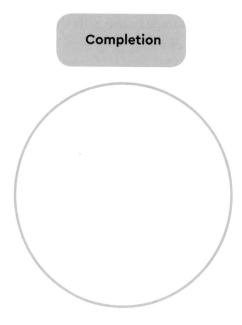

Completion

Do you long to completely fill in the circle? If so, try thinking about what you should do to meet that goal. Although you have examined them before, write down what values you will pursue, what things you will improve, and what new things you will create in your life in relation to completion.

▸   Core Values I Am Pursuing:

_____

_____

_____

_____

▶   Things to Improve:

▶   Things to Create:

Seeking Your True Self

Living the life others expected of them instead of living true to themselves—this was what many people regretted in the moment of death. What is a life that is true to oneself? To know that, we first have to know what the "self" is.

The true self is not external things. It is not your name, your body, or your thoughts. It is not your knowledge or experience, and not the things you possess. It is not your successes or your failures. Your true self is the essence of your being that is self-existent beyond all those external, artificial values. Other things that are not true self but perceived as "me"—that is ego.

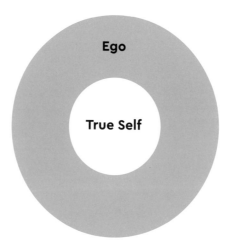

Have you ever felt your true self? Have you ever had the feeling, "This is the real me"? If so, describe the moment you felt that way and what it was like.

What self is now leading your life? Is it your true self? Is it your ego, things like your ideas, emotions, and desires? Or is it the expectations of others, the information you've received from those around you? Or some combination of them? Reflect on the nature of the main voices driving your life and write down your thoughts.

_____

_____

_____

_____

_____

Expressed another way, the true self is the "soul." The soul is not simply a theoretical concept. It is energy existing in our chests, and we can detect it through feelings.

Close your eyes and gently relax as you breathe in and out of your chest. Try to "feel" your chest. With your mind's eye, look into the center of your chest and try to focus on the sensations there. You may feel things like stuffiness, numbness, openness, warmth, or tingling, or things like anxiety, depression, love, peace, or joy. Write down what feelings you detected.

_____

_____

_____

_____

The feelings we detect in our chests reflect the condition of the soul energy found there.

- If your chest feels comfortable and warm, it means that the energy of your soul is awake and relatively stable.

- If your chest feels constricted or heavy, or if you have feelings like anxiety, depression, irritability, or worry, it means that the energy of your pure soul has withered; in contrast, the energy of your emotions is dominant.

- If you don't feel anything in your chest, it means that your sense for detecting your soul's energy is numb and that you are far from your true self.

Which of these three is closest to the feeling in your chest? Close your eyes and, focusing on your chest, try once again to feel the condition of your soul energy. Try to sense the feeling just as it is, without imagining or creating it. You can find the right solution when you've done honest watching. Write down what you felt.

No matter what condition you're feeling right now, there will be a reason for it. What do you think is the reason or cause for what you are feeling?

I would like to recommend some resources to help you awaken to the feeling and existence of your soul. Read my book *Bird of the Soul* or watch a video clip *Bird of the Soul Animated Storybook* on Live120YearsBook.com/resources.

What did you feel through the *Bird of the Soul* story? Did you have sympathy for the protagonist, Jay? In what parts of the story did you feel that way?

The state in which you feel that all is one, that is the state of a pure soul. As we grow up, though, we come to distinguish between mine and yours, between right and wrong, between doing well and making mistakes. As that happens, the energy of the thoughts, emotions, and desires inside us gradually takes up more space, and the pure energy of the soul is driven into a corner of our hearts.

When that suppression and frustration reach an extreme, these questions suddenly burst from inside us: "Is this living? What am I living for right now? What in the world is an authentic life?" That is an SOS signal sent to us by the energy of a soul long withered and abandoned.

Have you ever felt that SOS signal? When and how was it? What did you do when you felt the signal?

Whenever you feel the pure energy of your soul has been dimmed by the cares and worries of your daily life, you can clear away the energy of your thoughts and emotions that cover it and return your attention to it. I suggest these four steps for recovering your connection to your soul inside you.

Step 1. Feeling Your Soul

First you need to "feel" your soul. Being able to feel your soul means that you are connected and have started communing with it. Just concentrate on the feelings in your chest without thinking anything in particular at all. Try to sense your condition just as it is. If you're frustrated, then feel frustrated; if you get no feeling, then feel nothing at all.

Step 2. Questioning Your Soul

While feeling your chest, ask your soul, "What is it you really want?" You may not get an answer right away, but that's all right. Keep asking until you get an answer, either in words, images, or feelings.

Step 3. Detecting What the Soul Wants

Discern the feeling or voice of your soul to determine what your soul truly wants, what state it wants to achieve. Trust your ability to know what that is.

Step 4. Doing What Your Soul Wants

Apply and practice in your life what your soul wants according to the feeling or message of your soul. After taking action, try to sense your soul's feeling and satisfaction. Adjust your actions to maximize your soul's satisfaction.

Record what you experience in the following table as you practice feeling your soul and following your soul's desire every day for a week.

	Feeling/Message About What Your Soul Wants	What You Did, the Feeling of Your Soul After You Took Action
Day 1		
Day 2		
Day 3		
Day 4		
Day 5		
Day 6		
Day 7		

I've Decided to Live 120 Years Personal Workbook

Beginning a Life of Completion

The standard of completion is inside us; it's not determined by someone or something else. It is our soul. Our souls want to be illuminated, want to be liberated, and want to grow and be completed. Our soul energy doesn't want to be crumpled up in one corner of our hearts. It wants to be expressed, it wants to expand, and it wants to be shared. Living according to the feeling of what your soul desires, living centered on your own standard, your soul—that is the shortcut to completion.

For that to happen, the core value supporting the axis of your life should change—from success to completion! I'm not saying that success is bad, or that you shouldn't pursue success. Success is one means for achieving completion; but success itself should not be the purpose of life. If you want to achieve completion, you must make *completion* your core value.

What is it your soul ultimately wants to achieve? Is it success or completion? What will be your core value for the life your soul wants?

You don't need to wait until the second half of your life to choose to design your life from the perspective of completion. The younger you are when you do this, the better. It's enough to make completion the primary purpose of your life and to pursue and use "success" as a means for achieving that completion and for leading a beautiful life. Those who pursue success with completion as their core value will not be swept away by reckless competition, and they will use the success they've achieved as a good tool for completion.

Through the following exercise, try to feel how a life lived for the purpose of completion is different from a life lived for the purpose of success.

Make tight fists and take a deep breath, as deep as you can. Continue inhaling in that state until you can't anymore. Now relax your fists and breathe out. Write down how it felt when you kept inhaling and how it felt when you exhaled comfortably.

The period of success is a time for acquiring and accumulating. It's like holding our hands in tight fists and breathing in as much as we can. But no one can continue in that state. We have to relax our hands and breathe out. "Share and give" is the attitude of life in the period of completion.

Write down the things you've been pursuing while living for success and the things you should pursue when living for completion.

PARADIGM SHIFT

1ST 60 YEARS	2ND 60 YEARS

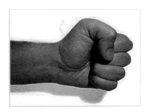 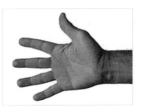

Living for Success	Living for Completion
• Pursuing external value • Competition necessary for achieving limited value • First-come, first-served race • The world is a battlefield where you have to fight and win	• Pursuing internal value • Competition unnecessary for achieving infinite value • A race where a winner's cup awaits everyone • The world is an honest garden where you reap what you sow
Things You Have Been Pursuing for Success	**Things You Will Pursue for Completion**

When life is viewed as a kind of circle, the first half is when people generally pursue success. But they feel that it's not at all clear what they should pursue in the second half. The opportunity has now come to complete the circle of life.

Now that you've practiced feeling the messages of your soul, look again at your values and goals. Assuming that half of the circle of your life has not been completed, how will you make the circle whole? Write down how you will live, what goals you will have, and what will serve as your center.

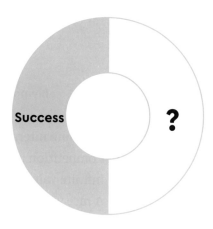

Value and Goal for Life: What do you want to achieve?

_____

_____

_____

Attitude Toward Life: How do you want to live?

_____

_____

_____

I've Decided to Live 120 Years Personal Workbook

Create a mission statement by combining the things you wrote above: your purpose in and attitude toward life. You may add details and update it as you go through this workbook, so just write down what you're thinking now, in a way that is comfortable for you. It can be just a few words, or it can be one or more sentences. Write down whatever comes to mind, without worrying about form.

My Mission Statement:

A path for completing ourselves and for completing life,
I think this is the truly human path that we, as humans, should walk.
—ILCHI LEE

HOW DO WE ACHIEVE COMPLETION?

Read Chapter 3 of *I've Decided to Live 120 Years* before starting this chapter.

We know what we are, but know not what we may be.
—WILLIAM SHAKESPEARE

Thinking About Death

There is an important milestone we should ponder on our way toward completion, along the path to a new life. That milestone is death.

The final settlement of accounts concerning the level of completion in our lives can only be done in the moment we face death. People who are satisfied with their lives generally experience tranquil deaths, while the deaths of those who have negative memories, awareness, or regrets about their lives are not so comfortable.

Have you ever seen a family member or friend facing death? If so, what feeling did you get from them? Did they look peaceful or troubled?

_____

_____

_____

_____

_____

Think about how that person looked immediately before death in connection with how they lived life. What kind of life did they live? Think about whether they accepted the adversities they experienced in life with a positive attitude or struggled with life's suffering.

_____

_____

_____

_____

_____

Have you ever thought about death? Describe the kinds of feelings or images that death brings to mind for you.

_____

_____

_____

_____

_____

_____

_____

Many people think that death is scary, painful, and sad. That could result from prejudices about death that have been influenced by their cultures, practices, and belief systems. Death is, in fact, an incredible blessing for our spiritual awakening. We feel an instinctual pull toward wholeness and eternity, transcending such limitations, because we are incomplete, finite beings. That's why I feel that death is a great design of the Creator, prepared for the completion of human life.

I learned from the *Sundo,* a traditional Korean system of mind-body training, to view death as the completion of the soul, not its end. In Sundo, *Chunhwa* is a type of death on the most beautiful and peaceful level that can be experienced by humans.

Translated literally, *chun* means "Heaven" and *hwa* means "become," so Chunhwa means to become Heaven, or heavenly transformation. Heaven here signifies both the Source of life and the heavenly nature that is a part of us—in other words, wholeness. Chunhwa points to the great cycle of actualizing completion within ourselves through the journey of our lives in this world and then the returning to the Source of life.

Understanding the Energy System
for Completion of the Soul

Chunhwa means a death in which completion of the soul is achieved. In Sundo, humans are believed to have a seed within them that allows them to reach completion. This seed of wholeness is the soul.

In Sundo, it is believed that our bodies contain a perfect energy system for achieving growth and completion of the soul.

Read about the energy system for completing the soul on pages 63 to 68 of *I've Decided to Live 120 Years*. Clarify what you've understood as you fill in the following blanks.

Location of Energy Center	Name of Energy Center	Name of Developed Energy State	Ideal Energy State
Abdomen			
Chest			
Head			

Experiencing Ki Energy

Your understanding of *ki* energy—the life energy that makes up all things—shouldn't remain only at the level of theory or knowledge. It's important that you feel it directly. Only then can you use and apply it in your daily life.

Have you had the experience of feeling ki energy? Everyone has a sense for feeling energy. This is because our minds and bodies are made up of energy. And our souls are made up of energy, too. If you want to feel your soul, all you have to do is feel ki energy. To feel ki energy, your thoughts and emotions must quiet down. Then your senses will be able to focus on the energy of your soul.

Follow these instructions to awaken your sense for feeling energy:

Sit comfortably in a chair or on the floor, and straighten your lower back. Place your hands on your knees, palms facing upward. Relax your neck and shoulders and release the tension throughout your body. Calm your mind. Take a deep breath, then slowly exhale. Release any remaining tension out of your body as you exhale.

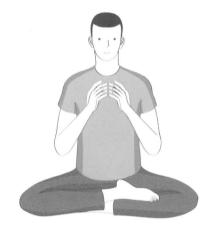

Now bring your hands in front of your chest and tap the tips of your fingers together. Do this for about 30 seconds, then slowly move your hands so that your palms face each other with about two inches between them.

Close your eyes and try to get the feeling that your hands are hanging in empty space. Imagine energy filling the space between your hands. That energy flows between your hands like fog or clouds. Picture energy filling the space between your hands and shining brightly.

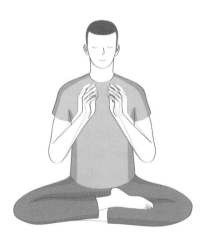

Now, very slowly, repeatedly move your hands a little apart and then back together, alternately expanding and contracting the space between them. Your hands gently push against and then pull away from each other, like a butterfly slowly flapping its wings. Continue repeating this movement until you get a feeling of magnetism between your hands.

How Do We Achieve Completion?

Try to sense what feelings you get in your hands. You might feel heat or a tingling sense of electricity in your hands, and you might get a feeling of magnetism or volume, as if there is a balloon between your palms. Those feelings are amplified as you continue to concentrate and pay attention to even subtle sensations.

Slowly lower your hands onto your knees. Take a deep breath and, exhaling slowly, open your eyes.

To further your understanding, watch the Energy Sensitizing Meditation video on Live120YearsBook.com/resources.

Did you feel energy through this training? Do your body and mind now feel more comfortable and relaxed than they did before? Describe what you felt, including even small sensations.

You don't need to be disappointed if you couldn't definitely feel ki energy just now. We are not familiar with focusing inward, because we are tense and live so much in our thoughts and feelings, and because our senses are generally turned outward. Even tiny sensations are good; if you continue to repeat the exercise, focusing on those feelings, you will be able to develop your energy sense. Remember that everyone has that sense, and keep trying to use it. It can be effective to try this practice after relaxing your body and mind through stretching or gentle exercise, sweeping the tangled thoughts from your head.

I've Decided to Live 120 Years Personal Workbook

Feeling Jungchoong, Kijang, and Shinmyung Energy

It is true that considerable focus, effort, and time are required to experience an energy state of *Jungchoong*, *Kijang*, and *Shinmyung*—the three steps of energy completion. I'll teach you a simple method of energy meditation that allows even beginners to get a taste of what that state is.

Sitting in a meditative posture, straighten your lower back and close your eyes. First, do the energy-sensitizing training described previously. As you concentrate on the space between your hands, gradually amplify the energy field there.

Now slowly bring your hands in front of your lower dahnjon, the energy center in your lower belly. Turn your hands so that both palms face your abdomen. Imagine an energy field being projected from your palms into the center of your lower abdomen.

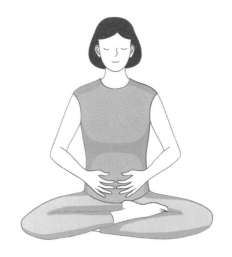

Now slowly and repeatedly move your hands away from and then closer to your abdomen. Feel and visualize the energy field between your palms and your abdomen gradually being amplified. Hold your palms still in front of your abdomen and send energy into the abdomen. Imagine energy filling your abdomen as you repeat to yourself, "Jungchoong, I'm being filled with jung energy."

After doing Jungchoong training for a while in this way, slowly bring your palms up in front of your chest. Imagine energy coming from the palms of your hands and entering your chest, your middle dahnjon system. Imagine the soul energy in your chest being activated.

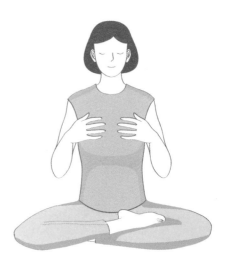

Now move your hands out from your chest and then bring them back again, slowly and repeatedly. Feel and visualize the energy field between your palms and chest gradually being amplified. Hold your palms still in front of your

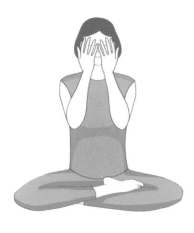

chest and send energy into it. Imagine energy filling your chest as you repeat to yourself, "Kijang, ki energy is growing more mature."

After doing Kijang training for some time in this way, slowly bring your palms in front of your face. Imagine healing your face with the energy coming from your palms. As you continue sending energy into your face, wear a big smile, stretching your facial muscles outward as much as possible. Stretch any of your facial muscles that are tense, one by one focusing on your forehead, eyebrows, cheeks, chin, nose, ears, and eyes.

Now hold your palms in front of your forehead, sending energy into it. Imagine bright energy coming from your palms into your upper dahnjon system, awakening the third eye, pineal gland in the center of your brain.

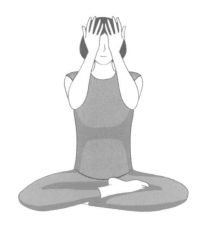

Bring your hands to the sides of your head. Moving your hands alternately away from and then closer to your head, feel the energy field between your head and your hands. Then hold your hands still and imagine energy coming from your palms into your brain. At this time, imagine the energy in your brain being activated and growing brighter as you repeat to yourself, "Shinmyung, shin energy is growing brighter."

After doing Shinmyung training for some time, slowly place your hands on your knees. Try to sense the energy coming from your lower dahnjon, middle dahnjon, and upper dahnjon. Now spend some time breathing and meditating as you imagine the energy system of your whole body being activated and circulating.

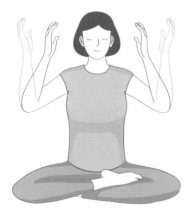

When you've finished meditating, slowly inhale and exhale. Open your eyes.

I've Decided to Live 120 Years Personal Workbook

What did you feel throughout this training? Describe what you felt.

Feeling of Jungchoong training (abdomen/vitality):

_____

_____

_____

_____

Feeling of Kijang training (chest/soul):

_____

_____

_____

_____

Feeling of Shinmyung training (face/brain):

_____

_____

_____

_____

If you've been able to get even a little feel for the process of Jungchoong, Kijang, and Shinmyung energy development, you are to be congratulated. Wanting to experience everything completely with one attempt, though, is unrealistic. Practice this method of energy meditation repeatedly.

My system of Body & Brain Yoga practice includes various methods for learning Jungchoong, Kijang, and Shinmyung, step by step and in depth. You may find a Body & Brain Yoga studio near you at BodynBrain.com.

Three Forms of Study

How can we pass through the stages of Jungchoong, Kijang, and Shinmyung to grow and complete the energy of our souls? A road map presented by Sundo points to using three kinds of study: the Study of Principles, the Study of Practice, and the Study of Living.

First, the *Study of Principle* is for awakening to the truth. Second, the *Study of Practice* is for feeling with your whole body your awakening to the truth; this is training for cultivating energy of body and mind. Third, the *Study of Living* is for practicing in your daily life your awakening to the truth.

The material of these three forms of study is your soul. They are about discovering the seed of the soul within you, causing the flower of your soul to bloom and produce fruit, and then sharing that fruit with many people. This whole process is made up of moments when the energy of your soul grows.

I believe that even those who don't know the concrete details of these three forms of study are practicing them in their own way in their daily lives if they are seeking to grow and cultivate themselves internally. For more detailed information on the three forms of study, see Chapter 4 in my book *Living Tao: Timeless Principles for Everyday Enlightenment*.

Look at the ways you are practicing these three forms of study in your own life. Think about what you should supplement and write that down here.

Three Studies	Things You Are Doing Now	Satisfaction Percentage	Ways to Supplement
Study of Principle			
Study of Practice			
Study of Living			

Chunhwa, Heavenly Transformation

When I describe the concept of Chunhwa, I often use as an illustration the story of the caterpillar's transformation. Just looking at its external appearance, nobody would guess that a crawling caterpillar will become a soaring butterfly. But hidden inside the caterpillar are factors allowing it to become a butterfly. In the same way, we humans have factors allowing us to attain Chunhwa.

The seed of attaining Chunhwa is our soul!

Take time to explore your feelings about Chunhwa as you watch the video on the caterpillar's transformation on Live120YearsBook.com/resources. Write down what you felt and understood.

Living a Soul-Centered Life

A soul-centered life is at the heart of living for Chunhwa. You grow and complete the energy of your soul in this way.

There's a principle for the growth of the soul's energy: your upper, middle, and lower dahnjons (the energies of your brain, heart, and belly) must be aligned and feel unified.

In the upper dahnjon (head), thoughts arise.
In the middle dahnjon (heart), emotions arise.
In the lower dahnjon (abdomen), actions arise.

Your thoughts (brain), feelings (heart), and actions (gut) shouldn't be separate; they should be one, and you should act with integrity. Your soul's energy is activated and grows when you are in a pure state, when your thoughts, feelings, and actions are one.

Examine where your thoughts, emotions, and actions are headed by considering the following:

Think of a particular problem you've been worrying about lately and write down what that problem is.

What is the direction of your thinking for solving that problem? To take care of it, are you thinking with your head about what you should do?

If you're actually acting in the direction you're thinking of, are you okay with that direction emotionally, too? Could it be that emotionally you'd like to pursue some other direction? Check whether your emotions agree with what you're thinking.

What actions are you taking right now to solve your problem? Or have you not yet acted? Check whether the direction of your actions is consistent with the direction of your thoughts and emotions.

Fill out the table below based on the checks you made on your thoughts, emotions, and actions.

What You Want	Direction for Solving the Problem	How the Direction Is Consistent or Inconsistent with Other Directions
What Your Thoughts (Head) Want		
What Your Emotions (Heart) Want		
Actions (Abdomen) Taken		

Do the problems you have cause you confusion or distress? If so, do you have a feeling for what is causing that confusion or distress? Confusion and distress occur when the directions of your thoughts, emotions, and actions are not consistent. You're confused and troubled inside because your thoughts, feelings, and actions are not aligned with each other.

What should you do in this case? How should you adjust the direction of your thoughts, emotions, and actions, and what direction should you follow?

_____

_____

_____

_____

When faced with such a situation, what will be the basis of your choice of direction? What is your reason?

_____

_____

_____

_____

You could do as your thoughts want, you could do as your emotions want, or you could simply act however your body and desire want. It's your choice and your freedom. No one can tell you to do this or that, choose for you, or force you to make a certain choice. That choice is yours to make, and the responsibility for that choice is also yours.

But I have a tip that will let you make the wisest choice if you want to live for the growth and completion of your soul: do what your soul wants, leading a soul-centered life.

For this, more than anything else, you have to recover the pure state of your soul and identify what your soul truly wants. Once you recognize what your soul wants, then your thoughts, emotions, and actions will start to align in the direction desired by your soul. At first it might be difficult to accept and it might take a lot of time, but once these three things align in the same direction that your soul wants, everything becomes simpler and clearer. "One Mind" is the power of the pure soul.

What's important is that your soul must first recover a pure state if you are to detect its definite direction. This is a state in which thinking and feeling have quieted and ceased, a state of peace and freedom without any attachments. To achieve this, it helps to do energy meditation for connecting with the energy of the soul.

Do the energy sensitizing training that was introduced on pages 65 and 66 in this workbook. Then bring your palms in front of your chest and do Kijang training for activating the energy of your soul. Imagine the energy coming from your palms amplifying the energy of your soul. When you feel that your soul energy has been sufficiently activated and purified, ask your soul about the problem that's bothering you, the one you wrote down earlier. Feel how your soul wants to solve that problem and write down what you feel.

Once you've identified the direction your soul wants to pursue for solving your problem, imagine your soul energy spreading from your chest to your head and lower abdomen. Visualize the energy of your head, chest, and abdomen aligning in a straight energy line. This is a process for integrating your thoughts, emotions, and actions centered on your soul. Now imagine the problem being resolved in the way your soul wants. Write down what you have felt during this process.

_____

_____

_____

_____

Internal conflict and confusion decrease when you are of one mind, centered on your soul. However, old habits may again cause your thoughts, emotions, and actions to become misaligned. It's important not to blame yourself at such times but to accept yourself as you are, and to make choices—again and again—in the way your soul wants.

When you live a soul-centered life for a while—one that unifies the directions of your thoughts, emotions, and action—the energy of your soul cannot help but grow. That is the shortcut to Chunhwa.

For the completion of your soul and Chunhwa, you must constantly ask your soul questions, make choices, and act. It's about making up your mind to save yourself instead of relying on anything external. I usually say this about Chunhwa: "Chunhwa is me saving myself." Realizing that your soul is the seed of wholeness inside you, you continue to develop it. When that wholeness grows and grows to take on nature's original form—in other words, when you are one with the fundamental life energy of the cosmos—you ultimately attain completion of the soul: Chunhwa.

Picturing an Enlightened Elder

As described on pages 72 to 74 of *I've Decided to Live 120 Years*, we can categorize three stages of human growth using the Korean word *eol*, which means "soul."

Growth Stages		Energy Stages		Maturity of Soul	Characteristics
Eorini (child)	Period of growth	Jungchoong	Physical power	Soul is young and small	Selfish, self-centered thinking, spontaneous behavior
Eoreun (adult)	Period of success	Kijang	Heart power	Soul has grown and matured	Sense of responsibility, tolerance, rational thinking and behavior
Eoreushin (elder)	Period of completion	Shinmyung	Brain power	Soul is illuminated, gaining wisdom	Broad tolerance, great love, bright wisdom

Which of the three stages are you currently in? Your soul could be mature even though you are young, or, conversely, your soul could be immature even though you are advanced in years. What is your growth stage physically, and what is the stage of your soul energy?

What do you need to improve in order to develop your soul energy in the future? Reflect on whether your thinking, emotions, words, deeds, and attitudes are mature. Write down in detail which areas you intend to improve and how.

_____

_____

_____

_____

Picture yourself as you will be when you are older. Do you picture an elder (*eoreushin*) with great love and bright wisdom? Describe who you want to be in your old age.

_____

_____

_____

_____

Our lives become works of art, not pain, when we know the law of Chunhwa.
— ILCHI LEE

CHAPTER 4

REFLECT ON THE FIRST HALF OF YOUR LIFE, DESIGN THE SECOND

Read Chapter 4 of *I've Decided to Live 120 Years* before starting this chapter.

What lies behind you and what lies in front of you,
pales in comparison to what lies inside of you.
—RALPH WALDO EMERSON

Reflecting on the First Half of Life

Renewal doesn't come automatically, and life doesn't change just because you're a year older. You can understand this even if you're only 30 years old. The years pass and the seasons change in accordance with the cycles of nature, but it is you who gives meaning to those changes and you who chooses renewal.

You can obtain wisdom and direction for that new choice by reflecting on your past. Your eyes of wisdom open when you start to see the things that you've been missing, the places where you've been inadequate, and the areas where you've made mistakes.

Look back again on how you've been living throughout life. As you reflect on your whole life, how do you feel about your past in general? Write down any specific scenes that stand out in your mind.

_____

_____

_____

_____

Powerful, impressive memories may come up, or you may detect only vague memories and feelings from your past. If you want to remember your history as times that were truly meaningful, not just wasted days gone by, what should you do?

You need to take time to look back on your life overall, time to reflect on what meaning those moments had for you and what lessons and growth they brought you.

Let's use two methods to reflect on your life. One is bringing to mind important events according to when they happened, and the other is introspection prompted by specific questions.

Can you guess how many hours you've lived so far? If you've lived for 30 years, it comes to about 260,000 hours; if 45 years, it's about 390,000 hours; and if 60 years, about 520,000 hours. Think about how many things have happened to you during all that time.

Looking back on your life may take quite a lot of time and may be hard to finish in one go. Take plenty of time to look at things carefully, in detail. If there isn't enough space to write it all down here, use the Notes pages at the back of this book.

When you look back on your life, don't simply stop at saying, "This thing happened to me." Reflect on what impact the event had on your life, and what lessons you learned through it.

Looking Back by Time Period

1. **In Early Childhood**

   ▸ Things That Happened:

   _____

   _____

   _____

   ▸ Personal Relationships:

   _____

   _____

   _____

   ▸ Lessons Learned:

   _____

   _____

   _____

2. **In Elementary School**

   ▸ Things That Happened:

   _____

   _____

   _____

▶ Personal Relationships:

_____

_____

_____

▶ Lessons Learned:

_____

_____

_____

3. **In High School**

▶ Things That Happened:

_____

_____

_____

▶ Personal Relationships:

_____

_____

_____

▶ Lessons Learned:

_____

_____

_____

4. In My 20s

▸ Things That Happened:

_____

_____

_____

▸ Personal Relationships:

_____

_____

_____

▸ Lessons Learned:

_____

_____

_____

5. In My 30s

▸ Things That Happened:

_____

_____

_____

▸ Personal Relationships:

▸ Lessons Learned:

6. In My 40s

▸ Things That Happened:

▸ Personal Relationships:

▸ Lessons Learned:

7. In My 50s

▸ Things That Happened:

_____

_____

_____

▸ Personal Relationships:

_____

_____

_____

▸ Lessons Learned:

_____

_____

_____

8. After 60s

_____

_____

_____

_____

_____

_____

Looking Back on Significant Moments

1. What things have I achieved in my life?

2. When was I most joyful?

3. When were things most trying?

4. How did I overcome hardship in those trying moments, and what did I learn through them?

5. What moments in my life do I regret?

_____

_____

_____

_____

6. When did I do things that made me feel proud and that I found rewarding?

_____

_____

_____

_____

7. What momentary choices became opportunities that changed my life?

_____

_____

_____

_____

8. What values did I try to remain true to throughout my life?

_____

_____

_____

_____

9. What helped me remain true to those values?

10. What got in the way of my remaining true to those values?

11. What life goals have I had so far?

12. What motivated me to establish those goals?

13. Which of my life goals have I achieved?

14. Which goals have I failed to achieve?

15. Who has had a great impact on my life so far and in what way?

16. Whom have I considered precious and want to express my gratitude to?

17. With whom do I have emotional issues that I need to resolve and why?

_____

_____

_____

_____

_____

18. What specific things have I really wanted to do but couldn't?

_____

_____

_____

_____

_____

Which method of questioning were you more enlightened by, looking back on the different periods of time in your life or examining your life's significant moments and goals? Why was it more helpful?

_____

_____

_____

_____

_____

I've Decided to Live 120 Years Personal Workbook

Finding Lessons in the First Half of Life

Looking back on your life and writing things down may cause you to experience new feelings or realizations. What did you feel or learn in that process?

_____

_____

_____

_____

What would you like to say to thank, comfort, and encourage yourself for your hard work in the life you've lived so far?

_____

_____

_____

You are looking back on your life in order to gain the wisdom to make your remaining time more fulfilling and meaningful. For that, you need a process for editing and reinterpreting the things that have happened to you in a way that contributes to your future life. In other words, I'm telling you to interpret your past suffering, hurts, and despair from a new perspective—one that won't get in the way of your future life. Don't stop at thinking, "These things were hard for me." Instead, resolve to think, "These things were hard for me, but I learned something through that hardship, and this is how I should live and think in the future."

Read the story of someone who lived such a life, Viktor Frankl, introduced on pages 84 and 85 of *I've Decided to Live 120 Years*. Write down what his story makes you feel and what you learned.

_____

_____

_____

_____

You, too, have probably had painful moments. And if you compared them with what Viktor Frankl went through, you may have gotten some comfort for your own suffering, realizing that it was really small in comparison. But whether suffering is great or small, it feels huge to the person experiencing it.

Let's now practice extracting life lessons from our painful memories.

Bring to mind the most difficult, painful memory in your life. Try to describe when it happened, the pain you felt then, and how negative your thoughts and emotions may have become.

_____

_____

_____

_____

What was your view of yourself and the world at that time? Certain people, when in pain, find things so hard that they say God is unfair or blame it on fate. They may even find themselves anguishing over questions such as, "Is this suffering all there is to life? What meaning does such a life have?" What about you?

How did you overcome or get past those difficult moments? If you gained any realizations or life lessons through those painful experiences, what were they?

When suffering moments of excruciating pain, we end up thinking harder and more earnestly about the true meaning of life. As the years go by, we come to realize that those painful times were opportunities that added depth and maturity to our inner world.

There may even be people who have never experienced trying or painful moments. But you can't necessarily say that you've lived well just because your life has been free of any great suffering. People generally experience greater inner maturity through pain. In moments of suffering, we face the stark reality of life without rose-colored glasses, and we dig deeper to find the true meaning of life.

Reflect on what meaning your moments of suffering have had and what impact they have had on your life. Look for whether there were inevitable reasons for them to happen.

_____

_____

_____

_____

Try using the following phrases to edit and reinterpret your painful past for a better life in the future:

- This happened to me:

_____

_____

- This is how I choose to think of what happened to me now:

_____

_____

What's important is to realize that you have created your life so far. Those who think that their current condition was not made by themselves but by their environment and situation can't choose and take responsibility for their own futures.

Make up your mind to think this way: "However I've been living, it has been my life and no one else's." Try to express that attitude in writing.

Have sincere gratitude for your own life's story and for all the places and people who have appeared as characters in it. Try to express that gratitude by writing it in your own words.

More than anything else, love and be grateful to yourself for making it through all those moments to arrive where you are now. Try to express that attitude in your own words.

We can never turn back the clock. All we have to do is gratefully accept the things that have worked out well and honestly acknowledge and learn from our foolish mistakes. We must never be discouraged or hold ourselves in contempt. We can't exert the energy to start over in the second half of our lives if we blame ourselves this way. Calmly reflect on the tale of your life thus far, but draw hope and enthusiasm from it. Let it be the source of new energy for the story of the life that you will create in the future.

Write down what you have felt and what you have resolved to do after reflecting and meditating on this.

Designing the Second Half of Life

The earlier we start designing the second half of our lives, the better. As early as our teen years, it's desirable for us to understand that life is a process of self-completion and that success is merely one stage—not the only one—in that process. By the time we're in our 50s at the latest, we should definitely have a direction for our old age so that we can prepare for the life we've chosen.

Many people spend their old age without any detailed plan for the second half of their lives, only to regret it later.

The confession of a 95-year-old on pages 89 and 90 of *I've Decided to Live 120 Years* is the story of Dr. Seokgyu Kang, founder of Korea's Hoseo University. Write down what you felt after reading this passage.

To design the second half of your life, what you should do first is to discover what life you really want to live. Once you have the great central axis in place, you can get into designing the details for making that life a reality.

Close your eyes and ask yourself what purpose or direction you truly want to pursue. Ask yourself what's in your *heart*, not in your head. Find what it is that your soul earnestly wants in your heart and what kind of life will bring real joy to your soul, beyond the answers set by the world. Write down the answer you've found.

The Life I Want:

_____

_____

_____

Once you've found your life's goal and direction, picture in detail what you should do to achieve it.

Close your eyes again. Now imagine your old age. What does your old age look like, and how are you living it? Where are you living, and what are you doing? What are you doing that makes you really happy? After taking plenty of time for deep meditation, try to describe in writing just what you saw and felt. You might also draw a picture of the life you envision.

_____

_____

_____

_____

_____

_____

In the picture of the future you imagined through your meditation, did you find what you want to do going forward? Do you feel happiness and satisfaction in that picture? Or does that image feel like it's not enough?

For now, think of this as having drawn a basic schematic for your life design. Just as an architect keeps upgrading and adding detail to his or her design until he or she is happy with it, continue to enhance your own design for the future. As you go through this workbook, your design for the future will take on more detail.

Providing for Your Own Health, Happiness, and Peace

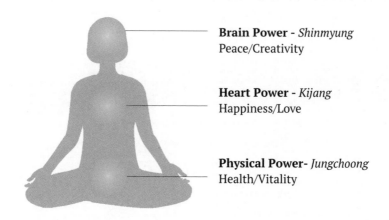

Brain Power - *Shinmyung*
Peace/Creativity

Heart Power - *Kijang*
Happiness/Love

Physical Power- *Jungchoong*
Health/Vitality

THREE TREASURES OF THE BODY, THE DAHNJON SYSTEM

Everyone should keep this one precept in mind when designing the second half of a life centered on the value of completion: you have to create your own health, happiness, and peace; you cannot rely on someone else to provide them.

Think about it. How could you hope to live a happy and beautiful life in old age by relying on your external environment—on other people or systems—for your health, happiness, and peace?

Are you healthy, happy, and peaceful now? Are you self-sufficient in these things, or do you tend to rely on your external environment for them? How many points out of 100 would you give yourself for each of them?

Am I healthy? _____ points

Do I provide myself with my own health? _____ points

Am I happy? _____ points

Do I provide myself with my own happiness? _____ points

Am I peaceful? _____ points

Do I provide myself with my own peace? _____ points

There's no need to be disappointed if your scores are low. You always have hope, because health, happiness, and peace are definitely variable and achievable, and because they are energy phenomena arising in your body.

In the following chapters, let's work in detail on health, happiness, and peace.

In the workshops I lead, I'm in the habit of ending sessions with the following cheer. Shout this with lots of feeling, imagining your physical power, heart power, and brain power reaching an optimal state. You may think it's silly, but try it anyway and see what changes it brings to your mood and energy.

Healthy Body, Happy Heart, Power Brain, Yay!

Water flows where directed. Where will the water of your life flow?
—ILCHI LEE

PHYSICAL POWER IS LIFE— JUST MOVE

Read Chapter 5 of *I've Decided to Live 120 Years* before starting this chapter.

The reason I exercise is for the quality of life I enjoy.
—KENNETH H. COOPER

Checking My State of Physical Power

Physical power is life. Physical power is proportional to your life force, so improving your physical condition is the best way to activate your life force and extend your lifespan.

If you don't know where or how to begin designing your old age, try starting with physical power. When your body develops strength, your ambition naturally grows along with it, and you find that you have new ideas and new things you want to try. It's a good idea to find a concrete physical goal for the level of physical power you want to reach or an ideal model you can imitate.

As you look back on your life, create a graph of trends for your health/energy activation.

Health/Energy Activation

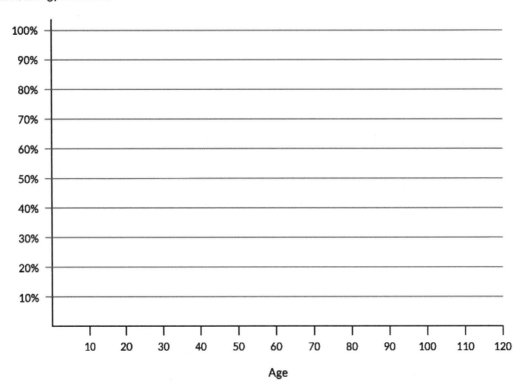

What do you want the condition of your health/energy activation to be going forward? Draw a graph above for your remaining time, showing your activation as you want it to be.

I've Decided to Live 120 Years Personal Workbook

Vital Age Test

The number of years you've lived tells you your physical age, but that number may not reflect your current state of health or energy activation. For that, I devised this test to calculate your Vital Age, which is the number of years you actually feel in terms of vitality, strength, range of movement, and lifestyle.

Check your current state of vital health based on the following 20 questions. Choose the most suitable answers for your personal condition, and then use the score sheet on page 111 to find your total.

1. Bring your feet together, clasp your hands in front of your body, and bend your upper body forward as shown in the following image. Be sure to keep your legs straight. How far do your hands reach?

    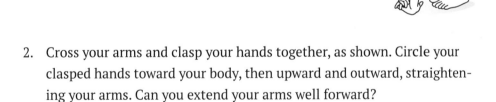

    A. Palms completely touch the floor.
    B. Fingers touch the floor.
    C. Fingertips touch the floor.
    D. Fingertips are lower than your knees.
    E. Fingertips are higher than your knees.

2. Cross your arms and clasp your hands together, as shown. Circle your clasped hands toward your body, then upward and outward, straightening your arms. Can you extend your arms well forward?

    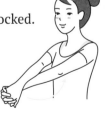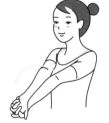

    A. Arms extend completely with fingers interlocked.
    B. Arms extend with elbows slightly bent.
    C. Arms extend to greater than 90 degrees.
    D. Arms extend to less than 90 degrees.
    E. Arms do not extend at all.

3. Extend your arms straight out to your sides, close your eyes, and raise your right knee so that it forms a right angle. Keep your left leg straight at this time. Hold this posture for 30 seconds. For how long can you hold a stable posture?

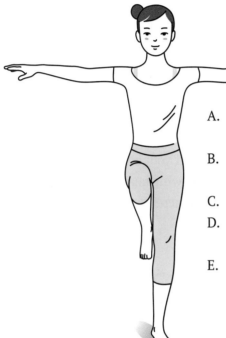

A. You maintain a stable posture for at least 30 seconds.
B. Your body is shaky, but your left sole doesn't come off the floor.
C. Your left sole comes off the floor several times.
D. You can't keep your balance, and your left foot keeps moving.
E. Your posture falls apart as soon as you stand on one leg.

4. Do the posture in Step 3, switching legs.

A. You maintain a stable posture for at least 30 seconds.
B. Your body is shaky, but your right sole doesn't come off the floor.
C. Your right sole comes off the floor several times.
D. You can't keep your balance, and your right foot keeps moving.
E. Your posture falls apart as soon as you stand on one leg.

I've Decided to Live 120 Years Personal Workbook

5. Starting from a seated position on a mat or the floor, stretch your arms forward, bring your legs together and raise them so that they form an angle of about 45 degrees with the floor, and tilt your upper body back to an angle of about 30 to 40 degrees, as shown in the following image. How long can you hold this posture?

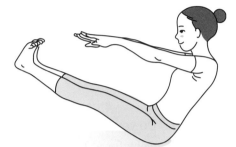

   A. More than 2 minutes
   B. 1 to 2 minutes
   C. 30 seconds to 1 minute
   D. Less than 30 seconds
   E. Difficult to hold posture at all

6. Do push-ups in the following posture. How many can you do continuously while maintaining this posture, bending your elbows to 90-degree angles?

   A. 21 to 30
   B. 11 to 20
   C. 6 to 10
   D. 5 or less
   E. None

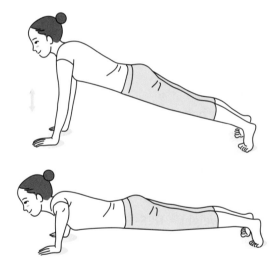

7. Stand up straight and relax your shoulders while looking into a mirror. Are your shoulders even?

   A. They are even.
   B. One side is slightly higher.
   C. One side is definitely higher.

8. When you sit in a chair, do you usually have your back and shoulders straight and open?

    A. Always
    B. Often
    C. Occasionally
    D. Rarely
    E. Never

9. Do you exercise regularly to manage your health? How many times per week for at least 30 minutes?

    A. 5 to 6 times
    B. 3 to 4 times
    C. 1 or 2 times
    D. Occasionally, when I think of it
    E. Almost never

10. What is your body mass index (BMI)? You can find this number by searching the Internet for a BMI calculator and entering your height and weight.

    A. Underweight = <18.5
    B. Normal weight = 18.5–24.9
    C. Overweight = 25–29.9
    D. Case 1 obesity = 30–34.9
    E. Case 2 obesity = 35 or greater

11. It's hard to get up in the morning.

    A. Always
    B. Often
    C. Occasionally
    D. Rarely
    E. Never

12. You overeat or eat irregularly.

    A. Always
    B. Often
    C. Occasionally
    D. Rarely
    E. Never

13. Your physical activities are limited because of your weight or the condition of your joints, heart, and lungs.

    A. Always
    B. Often
    C. Occasionally
    D. Rarely
    E. Never

14. You have constipation, diarrhea, or irregular bowel movements.

    A. Always
    B. Often
    C. Occasionally
    D. Rarely
    E. Never

15. You smoke.

    A. At least one pack a day
    B. One pack every 2 to 3 days
    C. One pack per week
    D. Less than 3 years since you quit
    E. At least 3 years since you quit, or you never smoked

16. You drink alcohol until you are drunk.

    A. Almost every day
    B. 2 or 3 times a week
    C. About once a week
    D. About 1 or 2 times a month
    E. Almost not at all

17. Your activities are restricted by stress or anxiety.

    A. Always
    B. Often
    C. Occasionally
    D. Rarely
    E. Never

18. You take medication for a chronic illness.

    A. 10 or more kinds daily
    B. 6 to 9 kinds daily
    C. 4 to 6 kinds daily
    D. 1 to 3 kinds daily
    E. Do not take medication

I've Decided to Live 120 Years Personal Workbook

19. You have frequent headaches.

    A. Always
    B. Often
    C. Occasionally
    D. Rarely
    E. Never

20. You're tired even though you sleep or get rest.

    A. Always
    B. Often
    C. Occasionally
    D. Rarely
    E. Never

Score Sheet

Ques. #	A	B	C	D	F	Ques. #	A	B	C	D	F
1	5	4	3	2	1	11	1	2	3	4	5
2	5	4	3	2	1	12	1	2	3	4	5
3	5	4	3	2	1	13	1	2	3	4	5
4	5	4	3	2	1	14	1	2	3	4	5
5	5	4	3	2	1	15	1	2	3	4	5
6	5	4	3	2	1	16	1	2	3	4	5
7	5	3	1			17	1	2	3	4	5
8	5	4	3	2	1	18	1	2	3	4	5
9	5	4	3	2	1	19	1	2	3	4	5
10	3	5	3	2	1	20	1	2	3	4	5

Results: Vital Age

81–100 Points: 20s–30s

Your flexibility, balance, and muscular strength are well developed and you have good lifestyle habits, so you're physically very healthy. Continue to maintain your present health.

51–80 Points: 40s–50s

You need to reflect on and improve your lifestyle habits. Your physical age could become 20 years younger than it is at present, depending on how you manage yourself from now on.

20–50 Points: 60s–70s

You don't get nearly enough exercise. You need to develop a habit of exercising in your daily life and work hard to take care of your body.

Overview of American Health Status

The obstacles many people face were driven home for me when I saw statistics on the status of health and healthcare in the United States. Currently, 87 percent of U.S. adults over the age of 65 have at least one chronic illness, while 68 percent have two or more. In comparison, 33 percent of adults over 65 in the United Kingdom and 56 percent in Canada have two or more chronic conditions.

U.S. OLDER ADULTS HEALTH STATUS

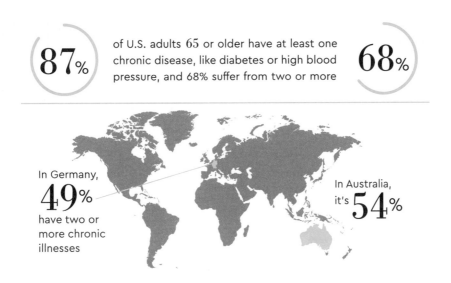

87% of U.S. adults 65 or older have at least one chronic disease, like diabetes or high blood pressure, and 68% suffer from two or more **68**%

In Germany, **49**% have two or more chronic illnesses

In Australia, it's **54**%

Source: The 2014 Commonwealth Fund International Health Policy Survey of Older Adults

To treat their illnesses, Americans rely heavily on medications—more than any other nation in the world. Although the United States holds just five percent of the world's population, it consumes 75 percent of its prescription drugs.

Overall, the United States spends more money on healthcare per capita than any other country ($9,507 per capita GDP in the United States vs. $3,763 per capita on average in Organization for Economic Co-operation and Development (OECD) countries in 2017). Unfortunately, healthcare costs can be too much for some individuals.

AVERAGE PER CAPITA HEALTHCARE COSTS IN OECD COUNTRIES

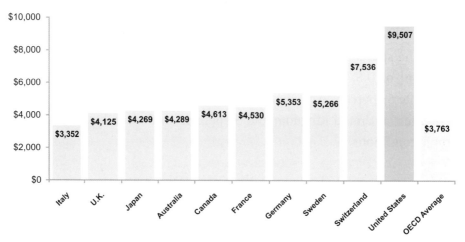

Source: OECD Health Statistics 2017 (Data are for 2015 or latest available)

According to one Harvard University study, healthcare spending accounts for 62 percent of bankruptcies in the United States. Among those who filed for bankruptcy due to medical expenses, 72 percent even had health insurance (source: *Huffington Post*, May 24, 2015). Health spending doesn't guarantee long life. Out of 224 countries, the United States ranks 31st in life expectancy in 2015.

LIFE EXPECTANCY VS. PER CAPITA HEALTHCARE SPENDING

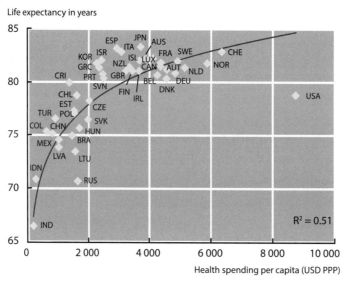

Source: OECD Health Statistics 2013

I've Decided to Live 120 Years Personal Workbook

According to a 2010 report by the Centers for Disease Control and Prevention:

38% of U.S. adults are obese.

17% of U.S. teenagers are obese.

44% of Americans will be obese by 2030.

Being overweight is a national health issue that affects the largest population (67 percent), forms the foundation for many other diseases and illnesses (such as Type 2 diabetes, heart disease, stroke, osteoarthritis, respiratory problems, cancers, and emotional disorders), and is the second most common cause of death next to smoking.

OBESITY RATES BY COUNTRY

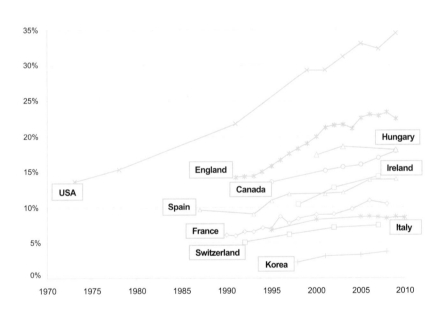

Source: OECD Obesity Update 2012

Checking Your Exercise Habits

Ultimately, all diseases share a single root. They always arise from blockage in the flow of energy, preventing an organism from accessing its original, natural healing power. Conditions causing most symptoms recover with time if you release blockages and restore good blood and energy circulation. Although we can't do anything about some factors, including genetics, others can be managed.

If you grow closer to your body, you can't help but grow more distant from hospitals and pharmacies. People who go to hospitals and pharmacies usually keep returning to them every time they feel ill. But we shouldn't rely on hospitals or medications every time we hurt a little. We should work to develop our own physical condition, telling ourselves, "When it comes to my body, I am the primary doctor." With will and effort, you can live a long, youthful, healthy life.

Exercise is truly a supplement that has a powerful effect. It's an exceptional method for enhancing life expectancy, health, and energy levels.

The World Health Organization recommends that adults should do at least 150 minutes of moderate-intensity aerobic physical activity or 75 minutes of vigorous-intensity aerobic physical activity throughout the week. Increasing the amount of exercise just a bit, though still falling below the suggested 150-minute mark, decreased the risk of premature death by 20 percent, and exercising exactly 150 minutes per week decreased that risk by 31 percent. Exercising 450 minutes per week (7.5 hours) decreased the risk of premature death by 39 percent. At any amount beyond 450 minutes, the risk plateaued.

Examples of Different Aerobic Physical Activities and Intensities

Moderate Intensity

- Walking briskly (three miles per hour or faster, but not race-walking)
- Bicycling slower than 10 miles per hour
- Tennis (doubles)
- Ballroom dancing
- General gardening

Vigorous Intensity

- Racewalking, jogging, or running
- Swimming laps
- Tennis (singles)
- Aerobic dancing
- Bicycling 10 miles per hour or faster
- Jumping rope
- Heavy gardening (continuous digging or hoeing, with heart rate increases)
- Hiking uphill or with a heavy backpack

How diligently are you exercising these days? Try to calculate how many times and how many total minutes you exercise per week. A general rule of thumb is that two minutes of moderate-intensity activity counts the same as one minute of vigorous-intensity activity.

	Exercise List	Moderate-Intensity Exercise Time	Vigorous-Intensity Exercise Time
1			
2			
3			
4			
5			
6			
7			
Total Time			

Calculate how much more or less you exercise than the recommended minimum of 150 minutes of moderate-intensity exercise per week. If you exercise less, write down how much you want to increase your exercise in the future and how you want to do it.

Even in terms of finances, exercise is the greatest preparation for old age. Becoming healthier is a way to avoid becoming poorer. By using your own body to heal your body on a daily basis, you can reduce or eliminate your need for medical treatment.

About how much have you been spending, on average, in medication and medical fees over the last several years? Has this amount increased or decreased over what it was when you were young? What is the reason for that? What will you do to reduce such costs?

Read the story of cyclist Robert Marchand, introduced on pages 105 and 106 of *I've Decided to Live 120 Years*. What did you feel as you read the story?

Proclaim to yourself, "I will protect my health." Close your eyes and, after resolving to provide for your own health, picture yourself in your old age, healthy and vigorous. How does that make you feel?

Give yourself hope and encouragement as you picture your healthy old age. Better late than never!

In the following pages, I'll introduce three kinds of opportunistic exercise to work into your daily life whenever you get the chance.

Experiencing One-Minute Exercise

For One-Minute Exercise, once every hour do a minute of moderate to vigorous exercise that effectively works your muscles and raises your heart rate in a short period of time—such as push-ups, squats, sit-ups, jumping jacks, jumping in place, and bear walking. If you cannot do this type of exercise, try a gentler form such as stretching, yoga, or tai chi. Choose exercises that work for you and make you happy.

Our body is designed to get better when we move. Sitting too long decreases circulation, interferes with oxygen and blood supply, creates stress, and weakens the skeletal structures and their supportive muscles.

Recent studies found that a sedentary lifestyle substantially contributes to major health concerns, including heart disease, high blood pressure, diabetes, cancer, and premature death.

Does One-Minute Exercise Really Work?

According to a sophisticated new study of interval training conducted by scientists at McMaster University in Hamilton, Ontario, 60 seconds of strenuous exertion proved to be as successful at improving health and fitness as 45 minutes of moderate exercise. The study researchers boiled down their findings to this simple message: "Stand up, sit less, move more."

Let's look at how much exercise you end up doing in total if you do One-Minute Exercise 12 times a day, from 9 AM to 8 PM, for one week:

- **Moderate One-Minute Exercise:** 12 minutes per day × 7 days = 84 minutes
- **High-Intensity One-Minute Exercise:** 12 minutes per day x 2 × 7 days = 168 minutes
- **Half High-Intensity, Half Moderate One-Minute Exercise:** 126 minutes

This amount of exercise covers most of the recommended minimum of 150 minutes of exercise per week. Of course, you'd get a greater effect if you exercised for at least 10 minutes at a time, but One-Minute Exercise has another effect: it can break the habit of continuous sitting.

Even if you exercise at a fitness center four or five times a week, if you spend most of your day in a chair or on a sofa, you will experience the "active couch potato" effect that comes from sitting for a long time.

Have you heard of "Sitting Disease"? It's a term coined by the scientific community that is commonly used when referring to metabolic syndrome and the ill effects of an overly sedentary lifestyle. According to Dr. James Levine, a medical director and obesity researcher at the Mayo Clinic and Arizona State University, "Sitting is more dangerous than smoking, kills more people than HIV, and is more treacherous than parachuting. We are sitting ourselves to death."

All right, now, that's enough sitting. Let's get up and try doing some One-Minute Exercise. Before your begin, write down how you feel, both physically and mentally. Then write down how you feel after you do One-Minute Exercise of push-ups or squats.

Before:

_____

_____

_____

After:

_____

_____

_____

Which of the following effects do you feel?

1. Physical energy is enhanced.
2. Body is warmer.
3. Mind is lighter.
4. Focus is developed.
5. Level of passion is increased.

Write down about 10 exercises you will do regularly to add One-Minute Exercise to your daily life.

_____

_____

_____

_____

_____

_____

_____

_____

We have an app, **One Minute Change**, that makes it possible for everybody to easily work One-Minute Exercise into their daily lives. Try downloading the app on Google Play or the Apple App Store or at 1MinuteChange.com and using it on your smartphone now.

Change yourself by doing One-Minute Exercise for at least seven days or up to 21 days. Record when you do it and the total number of times you do it.

Day	9 am	10 am	11 am	12 pm	1 pm	2 pm	3 pm	4 pm	5 pm	6 pm	7 pm	8 pm	Total
Day 1													
Day 2													
Day 3													
Day 4													
Day 5													
Day 6													
Day 7													
Day 8													
Day 9													
Day 10													
Day 11													
Day 12													
Day 13													
Day 14													
Day 15													
Day 16													
Day 17													
Day 18													
Day 19													
Day 20													
Day 21													

As you do One-Minute Exercise each day, circle which of the following effects you feel, and write down how you feel physically and mentally before and after you exercise.

Effects

1. Physical energy is enhanced.
2. Body is warmer.
3. Mind is lighter.
4. Focus is developed.
5. Level of passion is increased.

Day	Effect	Detailed Feelings
Day 1	1 2 3 4 5	Before: After:
Day 2	1 2 3 4 5	Before: After:
Day 3	1 2 3 4 5	Before: After:
Day 4	1 2 3 4 5	Before: After:
Day 5	1 2 3 4 5	Before: After:
Day 6	1 2 3 4 5	Before: After:
Day 7	1 2 3 4 5	Before: After:
Day 8	1 2 3 4 5	Before: After:

I've Decided to Live 120 Years Personal Workbook

Day	Effect	Detailed Feelings
Day 9	1 2 3 4 5	Before: After:
Day 10	1 2 3 4 5	Before: After:
Day 11	1 2 3 4 5	Before: After:
Day 12	1 2 3 4 5	Before: After:
Day 13	1 2 3 4 5	Before: After:
Day 14	1 2 3 4 5	Before: After:
Day 15	1 2 3 4 5	Before: After:
Day 16	1 2 3 4 5	Before: After:
Day 17	1 2 3 4 5	Before: After:
Day 18	1 2 3 4 5	Before: After:
Day 19	1 2 3 4 5	Before: After:
Day 20	1 2 3 4 5	Before: After:
Day 21	1 2 3 4 5	Before: After:

Experiencing Longevity Walking

Longevity Walking involves aligning your feet in parallel—like the number 11—and pressing down through the *yongchun* (the energy point just below the balls of your feet), flexing all the way to the tips of your toes.

Now try to walk in this position, imagining that your body is connected from your yongchun points to the crown of your head. Imagine that the energy in your body is connected from your yongchun points to the crown of your head, stimulating your brain.

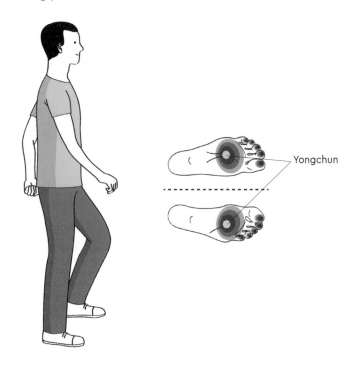

Yongchun

LONGEVITY WALKING FOR VITALITY AND ENERGY

1. Put your weight in your yongchun energy points.

2. Keep your feet parallel, like the number 11.

3. Press down through your yongchun points and squeeze your toes together.

4. Walk with the feeling of linking the soles of your feet to your brain.

Go outdoors and do Longevity Walking for 20 to 30 minutes. Before you begin, write down how you feel, physically and mentally. Then write down how you feel physically and mentally after doing Longevity Walking.

Before:

_____

_____

_____

After:

_____

_____

_____

Indicate which of the following effects you felt:

1. Physical energy is enhanced.
2. The soles of the feet and lower body are warmer.
3. Energy and blood circulation are enhanced.
4. Physical fatigue and pain are reduced.
5. Stress is reduced, and mood is improved.

Record how you change as you do Longevity Walking for at least seven days or up to 21 days. Circle which of the following effects you feel, and record how you feel physically and mentally before and after you do this exercise.

Effects

1. Physical energy is enhanced.
2. The soles of the feet and lower body are warmer.
3. Energy and blood circulation are enhanced.
4. Physical fatigue and pain are reduced.
5. Stress is reduced, and mood is improved.

Day	Time	Effect	Detailed Feelings
Day 1		1 2 3 4 5	Before: After:
Day 2		1 2 3 4 5	Before: After:
Day 3		1 2 3 4 5	Before: After:
Day 4		1 2 3 4 5	Before: After:
Day 5		1 2 3 4 5	Before: After:
Day 6		1 2 3 4 5	Before: After:
Day 7		1 2 3 4 5	Before: After:
Day 8		1 2 3 4 5	Before: After:

I've Decided to Live 120 Years Personal Workbook

Day	Time	Effect	Detailed Feelings
Day 9		1 2 3 4 5	Before: After:
Day 10		1 2 3 4 5	Before: After:
Day 11		1 2 3 4 5	Before: After:
Day 12		1 2 3 4 5	Before: After:
Day 13		1 2 3 4 5	Before: After:
Day 14		1 2 3 4 5	Before: After:
Day 15		1 2 3 4 5	Before: After:
Day 16		1 2 3 4 5	Before: After:
Day 17		1 2 3 4 5	Before: After:
Day 18		1 2 3 4 5	Before: After:
Day 19		1 2 3 4 5	Before: After:
Day 20		1 2 3 4 5	Before: After:
Day 21		1 2 3 4 5	Before: After:

Experiencing Belly Button Healing

Belly Button Healing is a quick, one-step, self-healing method of mindfully stimulating the belly button for gut and brain health, energy, and stress and pain relief.

The belly button is an important reflexology point at the center of your body for stimulating your intestines and brain at the same time. By applying Belly Button Healing two or three times a day for just five minutes, you can experience immediate stress and pain relief and also increased energy.

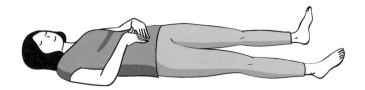

BELLY BUTTON HEALING

1. You can do Belly Button Healing lying down or standing up.

2. Relax your body and breathe comfortably for about one minute while focusing on your lower abdomen.

3. Press your belly button with the three middle fingertips of both hands rhythmically, repeatedly, and mindfully for about 100 to 300 repetitions.

4. After finishing, spend a couple of minutes focusing on your breathing, feeling your body more relaxed and refreshed.

 You can use a Belly Button Healing wand specially designed for the practice, for easier and more effective application.

For a detailed description of Belly Button Healing, visit www.BellyButtonHealing.com.

You'll find specific information there on the effects of this practice, read doctor recommendations, and watch many testimonial videos. You can also purchase Belly Button Healing products online.

Let's experience Belly Button Healing. First write down how you feel physically and mentally before doing the practice. After doing the exercise for three to five minutes, lie down and breathe slowly. Record how you feel physically and mentally after doing Belly Button Healing.

Before:

_____

_____

_____

After:

_____

_____

_____

Indicate which of the following effects you felt:

1. Tension and stress are relieved.
2. Breathing is deeper and more comfortable.
3. Pain is reduced.
4. Abdomen and lower body are warmer.
5. Vitality is enhanced.

Record how you change as you do Belly Button Healing for at least seven days. Circle which of the following effects you experience, and write down how you feel physically and mentally before and after you do the exercise.

Effects

1. Tension and stress are relieved.
2. Breathing is deeper and more comfortable.
3. Pain is reduced.
4. Abdomen and lower body are warmer.
5. Vitality is enhanced.

Day	Time	Effect	Detailed Feelings
Day 1		1 2 3 4 5	Before: After:
Day 2		1 2 3 4 5	Before: After:
Day 3		1 2 3 4 5	Before: After:
Day 4		1 2 3 4 5	Before: After:
Day 5		1 2 3 4 5	Before: After:
Day 6		1 2 3 4 5	Before: After:
Day 7		1 2 3 4 5	Before: After:
Day 8		1 2 3 4 5	Before: After:

Day	Time	Effect	Detailed Feelings
Day 9		1 2 3 4 5	Before: After:
Day 10		1 2 3 4 5	Before: After:
Day 11		1 2 3 4 5	Before: After:
Day 12		1 2 3 4 5	Before: After:
Day 13		1 2 3 4 5	Before: After:
Day 14		1 2 3 4 5	Before: After:
Day 15		1 2 3 4 5	Before: After:
Day 16		1 2 3 4 5	Before: After:
Day 17		1 2 3 4 5	Before: After:
Day 18		1 2 3 4 5	Before: After:
Day 19		1 2 3 4 5	Before: After:
Day 20		1 2 3 4 5	Before: After:
Day 21		1 2 3 4 5	Before: After:

In order to increase the state of your health/energy activation, it is important to find a concrete physical goal for the level of physical power you want to reach. Write down the number of times you have done each exercise in the table below for one minute. And make your goals of the number you want to increase in a month and three months later. You can add to the table if there are others exercises you would like to do.

Exercise	Current Number	Goal Number After One Month	Goal Number After Three Months
Squats			

When we manage our physical condition, we end up managing our time, emotions, and goals, and these come together as life management.
—ILCHI LEE

DISCOVER NEW SOURCES OF HAPPINESS

Read Chapter 6 of *I've Decided to Live 120 Years* before starting this chapter.

Happiness is not something ready-made. It comes from your own actions.
—DALAI LAMA

Checking Your Happiness

We can say that "happiness" is a general expression for the reason humans go on living. Is there a single person in this world who doesn't want to be happier? But many people go on living repetitive, unhappy lives, day in and day out, having forgotten to ask themselves, "Am I happy like this?"

Do you want happiness? If you want to be happy, stop for a moment and ask yourself, "Am I happy now?" If the answer you get is that you're not happy, then ask, "Why am I not happy?" Only one thing can give you a definite answer to this question: your soul, the true self in your heart.

If you want to find happiness, then you must have the courage to encounter your true self and question yourself. The soul in your heart will react, for the wellspring of happiness is in your heart.

Check your level of happiness and your tendencies regarding happiness through the following questions.

Ask yourself, "Am I happy now?" What answer do you hear in your heart? Write down what you feel.

_____

_____

_____

_____

_____

If you're happy, ask yourself why you're happy, or if you're unhappy, ask why you're unhappy. Why do you feel happy or unhappy? Write down your feeling and thought.

_____

_____

_____

_____

_____

_____

When do you feel happy? At what moments in your life do you usually feel happy? Provide concrete examples.

Everyone has his or her own thoughts about this: "To me, happiness is this." What do *you* think happiness is? Write down your definition of happiness.

To me, happiness is

Do you tend to wait for somebody else to make you happy, or for happiness to come to you when the situation surrounding you improves? Or do you try to find your own inner happiness? Write down your general attitude/tendency about happiness.

As you look back on your life, create a graph of trends for how happy/satisfied you have been at different times in your life.

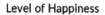

Level of Happiness

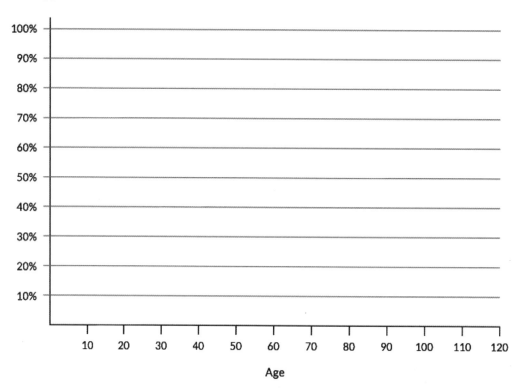

Age

What do you want the level of your happiness to be going forward? Draw a graph above for your remaining time as you want it to be.

I've Decided to Live 120 Years Personal Workbook

Identifying Why Your Aren't Happy

Generally, the first reason people feel they are unhappy is that they are unsatisfied with their environment. They have the sense that something is lacking.

What do you feel is lacking? In what areas do you need to be more satisfied in order to be happier? Write down what those things are.

Listed on the next page are conditions that people usually think are important for a happy life. Write down your degree of satisfaction in each area and your present situation and awareness.

Item	Satisfaction %	Your Current Situation and Awareness
Health		
Money		
Appearance		
Personal Relationships		
Work-related Relationships		
Achievement (work/ social activities)		
Past Experiences/ Memories		
Plans/Preparations for the Future		
Other Things You Want to Add		

By going over each item on the checklist, you have probably identified in a little more detail what you are satisfied and unsatisfied with. If you're unhappy because of your dissatisfactions, there are generally two solutions. One is to change your attitude in feeling that something is lacking. The other is to make up for the areas where you feel something is inadequate.

Reflect deeply on whether the lack you feel in these areas is a result of your own excessive expectation, attachment, or delusion. What did you feel?

Do you still have attachments to the things you're dissatisfied with? If so, try switching the way you think. Focus on what you have now, not on what you lack. Write down the things you have—for example, "I have a family that loves me and friends, like so-and-so and so-and-so. It's not a lot of income, but I have a job that lets me lead a stable life, and I have a body that I can move myself, without relying on others...." Write down even little things that you have been taking for granted. And try to feel gratitude for them. The more you write, the better.

You feel a little better, don't you, after writing down what you're grateful for? Don't you get a feeling of tranquil happiness? Happiness isn't some gigantic thing. If you just change your mindset, you'll find happiness there smiling back at you.

Setting aside your selfish desires and changing your mind is the quickest way to be happier, but there still could be times when you feel that your unsatisfactory environment gets in the way of your happiness. What should you do then?

If your environment is unsatisfactory, it's enough to try to change that environment so that you feel satisfied with it. It's about mastering your environment, directing and changing it yourself, not just blaming your surroundings for your dissatisfaction.

Keep in mind that although there are things you can change by your efforts, there are also things you cannot change, no matter how hard you work at it. If you try to change even the things you cannot change, that will inevitably move you away from happiness.

Are you working to change an environment you find unsatisfactory? What efforts are you making? Or are you just hoping your external environment will change, without putting much effort into making a difference? Write down your current situation and attitude.

You can, in fact, view most of the things you've been doing in your life as efforts to make your environment better. You've probably experienced a lot of hard things in that process. Look back on what attitudes you've had and on how you've dealt with things when you've encountered difficult situations.

Read the story of what I experienced at JFK airport in New York City on pages 148 to 150 of *I've Decided to Live 120 Years*. Have you ever encountered a great difficulty or obstacle? If so, write something about that situation and the bewilderment or confusion you felt.

_____

_____

_____

_____

_____

How did you deal with your situation? Did you overcome the difficulty, or were you discouraged by it? If you were able to get the better of it, did you give yourself some affirmation?

_____

_____

_____

_____

_____

The power to give yourself messages of affirmation and overcome problems even in difficult environments—that is the power of the soul.

Don't fear obstructions. It's difficult to break through a barrier if you think it is a thick wall. Based on the experiences of my life so far, obstacles are not thick walls; they are merely thin paper curtains that look thick on the outside. Push through, and they open up. Many people, though, are afraid and don't even think about breaking through those walls.

Wouldn't it be great if everyone could experience only good environments? That's not the way of the world, though. Due to limited values, it is natural that where there are winners, there are also losers, and if some are laughing, others are crying. The important thing is the perspective with which you look on the environment that has been given to you. Think of your environment, whether good or difficult, as a problem that has been given to you for the growth of your soul. Explore ways to achieve your soul's growth through it.

Think of the environment you're currently facing as a project you can use to develop the power of your soul. In the space below, write down the environments you evaluated earlier as giving you a low level of satisfaction. Reflect on what you have to learn through each of those environments and what issues you should resolve through them.

Decide whether you'll continue to be controlled by a difficult environment or will change your environment as an active creator. That change starts in your heart. I gave my brain a message of affirmation after losing my bags at a strange airport in a foreign land. In the same way, choose a positive message using "I" to overcome your difficult situation and write it down below.

With your eyes closed, repeat to yourself several times the affirmation you've chosen. Do this until your brain and soul react. Write down the feelings you had in your brain and soul when you gave them this affirmation.

For a week, after acting on the affirmation you've chosen, write down what you experienced. Keep repeating that message of affirmation. Do it until your habitual patterns of negative thinking change.

Discovering New Sources of Happiness

We often say that we are unhappy because of our unsatisfying environments. Could we really be happy, then, if we got the environment we wanted? There are many so-called "successful" people in the world who have all the conditions generally considered necessary for happiness. They aren't all happy, though. Why is that?

Even with a good house, car, and partner—commonly thought to be conditions for happiness—tedium and boredom are bound to come. Why? They have failed to discover something granting them true meaning and motivation in life, something that lets them live every day with heart-pounding passion.

What about you? Do you have something that gives your life meaning and motivation? If you do, what is it? If you don't, consider whether you've felt the need to find something like that and whether you have tried to discover it.

What are the sources of joy in your life right now? What are you doing when you feel joyful?

People usually feel joy when their needs are being satisfied. That includes the desire for food, sex, possession, and control. Satisfying such needs isn't wrong—in fact, people get a great deal of joy through these things. But if you continue to focus only on such joys and seek to alleviate life's tedium only through them, you're unlikely to gain opportunities to taste true joy, especially when you are older.

Besides the joys you have now, do you want to feel joy on another level? If you do, write down what you think that would be.

Pursuing new sources of happiness is like digging a new well. If the spring waters you used to drink no longer relieve your thirst, you need to dig another well for new sources of joy.

Are you working to dig a well of new joy? What kind of joy is it, and what efforts are you putting into it? Or, watching that old well drying up, are you waiting for someone to pour water into it or for the rains to come and fill it for you? Reflect on your current situation and attitude and write down your thoughts.

Don't just wait for someone else to bring you happiness, and don't just wait for your external environment to change. If you want to be happy, dig your own well of happiness. The well of true happiness is found inside you, and nowhere else. Remember: you are the only one who can find its source and dig for the spring of happiness within you.

Let me introduce three sources of joy that will quench your soul's thirst. If your life now is tedious and dull, I want you to drink from these springs of joy. You will taste a happiness that will leave your heart refreshed and full.

THE JOY OF HONGIK

The first spring is the joy of Hongik.

In the Korean word *Hongik*, *hong* means "widely," and *ik* means "to benefit." It speaks of doing things that widely benefit many people, not just me and my family. Hongik is a great love, a love that does not hope for reward.

Our souls are truly more joyful and freer when they have great love than when they cling to small love. This is because the energy of the souls in our hearts is so vast. That soul energy wants to flow out toward other people and the world. It wants to somehow be of help to them, even if it's only in little things, for then it can confirm the value of its existence. Doing what the true self wants, that is self-realization. The pure joy of the soul comes through such self-realization. That is the joy of Hongik.

Have you tasted the joy of Hongik? Have you ever helped someone out of a pure, spontaneous desire that didn't look for reward? If you have, when was that, and how did your heart feel then?

Only those who have practiced Hongik can taste its joys. For that, the process of digging their own well is necessary. What will you do to taste the joys of Hongik? Set up a short-term plan (perhaps for one month) and also a long-term plan.

Short-Term Plan:

_____

_____

_____

_____

Long-Term Plan:

_____

_____

_____

_____

After acting on your short-term plan this week, write down what you felt and experienced as a result.

_____

_____

_____

_____

THE JOY OF AWAKENING

The second spring is the joy of awakening.

"I think, therefore I am." As the words of Descartes suggest, the human, called *Homo sapiens*, is a thinking animal with high-level cognitive functions. Thinking is the moment when you awaken to your existence.

The deeper our thinking goes, the more we humans are naturally curious about the essence of existence and the principles of nature, biological life, and human life. Having that curiosity and wonder is the starting point for pursuing the joy of awakening. If you want to fill a tedious life with more meaning, then start by having curiosity.

Who am I? What is the meaning of human life? Such fundamental curiosity is good, and a curiosity that seeks to understand the meaning underlying the various personal relationships and twists and turns in your life is good, too. It's also good to approach this issue with interest in how your family, friends, and colleagues are living, what they're worried about, and how you might be able to help them. It's good to have curiosity about the small things, wondering "Why is the sky blue?" or "Why is the sunset red?"

Contemplating things as you go for a walk or taking a trip is good, meeting or contacting people is good, doing an Internet search is good, and going to a library or bookstore to read books is good. Having curiosity about yourself, others, and the world will fulfill your brain's intellectual needs and give your relationships and life greater color and richer flavor.

Have you tasted the joy of awakening? Have you ever given yourself over completely to solving some question—whether it's about the essence of life, the principles of nature and biological life, or personal relationships—and as a result experienced the joy of discovering the answer? If you have, try to describe what your situation was and the joy you felt then.

The joy of awakening begins with having questions and curiosity. Do you tend to be curious or incurious? Examine your tendencies.

If you lack curiosity, how do you want to develop your curiosity and about what? Are there things you want to take interest in, know, or study? Set up both a short-term plan and a long-term plan for doing this.

Short-Term Plan:

_____

_____

_____

_____

Long-Term Plan:

_____

_____

_____

_____

After acting on your short-term plan this week, write down what you felt and experienced as a result.

_____

_____

_____

_____

_____

THE JOY OF CREATION

The third spring is the joy of creation.

Human imagination and the creativity to turn imagining into reality are truly amazing. Creation is a privilege given to human beings and an ability every person has. We want to create something. Creation is an essential need of our brains. When we create, we experience genuine satisfaction and joy as our brains are activated.

It's good to taste the joy of expressing your inspirations through work, artistic activities, or hobbies, and it's also good to take care of the things you've been putting off in your life, to improve things that have been inconvenient, or to try challenging yourself with new things.

Remember these two principles of creation I'm suggesting:

First, there is no creation without action. No matter how good your thoughts or ideas may be, unless you act on them, nothing happens in reality.

Second, creation begins in you. Self-renewal—changing yourself to be new—is the beginning of creation and a steppingstone to greater creation.

Have you ever tasted the joy of creation? Do you remember a moment when you were inspired and created something new? Write down what you were doing then and how the joy of creation felt at that time.

Creation begins in you. How do you want to renew and change yourself? Set up both a short-term and a long-term plan.

Short-Term Plan:

_____

_____

_____

Long-Term Plan:

_____

_____

_____

Do you have a special project you would like to use to challenge yourself to lead a creative life? If you do, write down a short-term and a long-term plan.

Short-Term Plan:

_____

_____

_____

Long-Term Plan:

_____

_____

_____

I've Decided to Live 120 Years Personal Workbook

After acting on your short-term plan this week, write down what you felt and experienced as a result.

_____

_____

_____

_____

_____

_____

Are you worried because you're not happy? Happiness is not brought to you by others but something you create yourself.

If you can begin your day with excitement and end your day
in fulfillment and gratitude, that is happiness.
—ILCHI LEE

LET GO OF ATTACHMENTS TO FIND PEACE

Read Chapter 7 of *I've Decided to Live 120 Years* before starting this chapter.

Life is really simple, but we insist on making it complicated.
—CONFUCIUS

Checking for Peace of Mind

In old age, people aren't shaken up by much, because they do a good job of regulating their emotions and are less impulsive than when they were younger. This is due not only to a change in the older brain when people come to rely less on the happiness hormone dopamine, but also due to the learning and experience they've gained from all the storms of life.

This doesn't mean, however, that all factors causing disturbances of the mind completely disappear in old age. We need to open our mind's eye, watching for those factors, and we need to continue cultivating our inner world so we aren't affected by them.

Check your peace of mind through the following questions.

What do you think being at peace is? If you were asked to picture someone who is at peace, what would that look like? Describe the picture that comes to mind.

Is your mind at peace? How peaceful is it? Are you satisfied with the peace you feel?

My guess is that you're not always at peace but don't always lack peace of mind, either. What do you feel is the ratio between the times when your inner world is peaceful and the times when it's not?

I've Decided to Live 120 Years Personal Workbook

If you feel relatively peaceful now, you probably weren't always that way. Write down the changes of heart you've had that have brought you to the place where you are now.

If you feel relatively little peace right now, it's probably because something unresolved is still disturbing your mind. Watch your mind to see what it is, and write it down.

As you've lived your life so far, when did you feel very peaceful? Describe the situation and what your state of mind was like.

Find something that your imagined picture of a peaceful person has in common with the times when you've been at peace. What is it?

One thing that people who feel peaceful have in common is that no disturbances arise in their minds, and this is because they aren't attached to anything. That is the freedom of the soul.

Understanding Attachment

Let's think about this in reverse. If you're not at peace right now, it means your mind isn't free. Why? Because you are attached to something. That attachment causes disturbances in your mind, which keep you from being free.

You must be freed from those attachments to be more peaceful. For that, first you must honestly watch yourself just as you are, without adding or subtracting anything. It's important to accurately perceive what you are attached to and how strong that attachment is.

Take some time to examine and understand your condition frankly, based on the following questions.

Reflecting on Attachment to Wealth and Material Things

1. How important do you consider money, based on your criteria for evaluating people or value? Do you treat people who have a lot of money differently from people who have little? Bring to mind your actual experience with this, and write it down.

2. Do you tend to be greatly affected by situations involving financial losses or gains? Bring to mind your actual experience with this, and write it down.

3. Have you ever experienced mental suffering due to money or material things? Bring to mind your actual experience with this, and write it down.

4. When you were young, was your family wealthy or poor? What did your parents or family generally tell you about money?

5. When you were young, did you ever think, "I'm going to make a ton of money when I grow up"? How do you feel your environment or personal experiences have affected you in the formation of your ideas about money?

6. Do you believe you can design a future without scarcity if you earn money honestly and with integrity? Do you hope to create great profits through a one-time investment, or do you hope that great fortune will come your way?

7. What kind of emotional reaction do you experience when you see someone who is overly greedy for wealth and material things?

8. Do you tend to contribute and share materially with your family, the people around you, or social groups?

9. Do you feel relatively comfortable or uncomfortable about your present financial condition or your situation related to money?

I've Decided to Live 120 Years Personal Workbook

10. Do you think that attachment to wealth and material things contributes to a life lived for the growth and completion of your soul? What is your reason for thinking as you do? If the way you think about material things doesn't help, how do you want to improve it in the future?

Wealth and material things are not themselves a problem, because we definitely need them to live our lives. If we have a lot of material things, we have that many more opportunities to contribute to others. So if we use these things well, they can be good tools for the growth of our souls. The problem is attachment to them.

Excessive greed for wealth and material things is a problem, but being disgusted by people or situations where such avarice is at play is also a problem. Hating something too much, in fact, means that you are bound to it. Our minds finally find peace when we neither like nor dislike something too much. For then our minds are not disturbed by an attraction or aversion to things. Finding such a state of harmony and balance is a shortcut to peace of mind.

Reflecting on Attachment to Power and Prestige

1. Write down the social status or power you have now and the prestige you feel. Are you satisfied or dissatisfied with them? Why? How do you want your social status, power, and prestige to develop going forward?

2. Pursuing power is deeply related to the need for control. Do you feel joy and a sense of superiority when you control and dominate other people? Or do you feel defiant or inferior when you are instructed to do something by others or under their control? Write about your experience and emotional reactions related to this.

3. Pursuing prestige is deeply related to the need for recognition. Do you feel that you get enough recognition for your efforts at home or at work (in society)? Or do you feel that you don't get proper recognition for your efforts and true value? Write down what you feel about this, divided into two areas: home and work (society).

4. Look back on when you were young. Have you ever felt that you were mistreated or not properly recognized at home, at school, or among your friends? If you've had such experiences, write about what happened and what you felt then. And reflect on what influence such experiences have had on your life.

5. Did you tend to be very competitive when you were young? Have you ever been competitive in your dealings with even close friends because, more than anything, you wanted to be superior to them in your school grades or in an area you liked? Conversely, did you give up on competing altogether? Write down your disposition as a child regarding competition. Reflect on what influence such experiences have had on your life.

6. How strong is your competitiveness right now? Do you have a rival you are aware of at present? Who is it? What is your emotional reaction when you feel that this rival is ahead of you? Or do you tend to live without being very competitive?

7. Do you think that you should be more successful than your siblings or friends, and that you should work better and harder than your colleagues and get recognition for it? Is your personality such that you can't stand being behind others even in little things? Or do you choose to live comfortably because you have given up on or dislike competition?

8. Do you tend to be greatly influenced by how the people around you look at you or evaluate you? Do you consciously do things to look good to others? Have you ever hoped that other people would recognize you for some good deed you've done? Looking back on your experiences, write an answer for each of these questions.

9. Do you give yourself recognition, or do you criticize and constantly push yourself? Describe your attitudes or tendencies around self-recognition.

10. Do you think that attachments to power and prestige contribute to a life for the growth and completion of your soul, or not? Why do you think as you do? If something about your thinking doesn't help, how do you want to improve it in the future?

Beware of avarice for power and prestige; being disgusted by people or situations is, in fact, a disorder in the mind created by attachment. The problem is not power and prestige themselves, but the mind that is attached to them.

You need to let go of your attachments but also have the will to use your power as a tool for the growth of your soul. When it's used well, power can be a wonderful tool capable of helping people. If those in high positions use their power with a lofty, noble awareness, they will have a positive influence on many people.

The best way to resolve your obsession with power and prestige is to recognize yourself instead of hanging on to recognition that other people give you. The acknowledgment of your soul is greater recognition than anything else. Along with an inner feeling of pride, the greatest praise is a voice inside you saying, "Yeah, you did great!" Your soul recognizing and being satisfied with you is like Heaven recognizing you. That bright true nature, the soul within you, is Heaven.

Close your eyes and say something to yourself that acknowledges yourself. After doing this, write down what you felt.

Reflecting on Attachments to People You Like

1. Is there anyone you're attached to because you like them too much? Who is it? How is your attachment expressed? Has the other person ever reacted in a way that expressed dislike for your attachment?

2. What emotional reactions do you experience when the person doesn't meet your expectations? How do such emotions trouble and make things difficult for you? If you've had such an experience, write it down.

3. Have you ever attempted or strived to be free from your attachment to the other person? If so, what did you do? Why was it hard to let go of that attachment?

4. Have you experienced a similar attachment to another person as well? If so, when was it and who was it? What did the distress you experienced because of that attachment feel like, and what impact did it have on your relationship? What did you learn through that experience?

5. If you reflect on the experiences and lessons from your past, you will see your present attachments more clearly. Think about how you will apply what you learned from your past experiences to your present relationships to avoid repeating the same mistakes. Write that down below.

_____

_____

_____

_____

_____

_____

Liking someone too much is also an attachment. You might really like them, but they might not respond as favorably as you hope. There is no rule that says the other person has to like you as much as you like them. He or she has the freedom and right to choose, even if it means disliking you. Haven't you ever disliked someone who liked you? Try to acknowledge that the person you like may dislike you in that same way.

You might think that you're suffering because of the other person, but in fact, you're suffering because of your attachment. The quickest way to be at peace is to clearly see and let go of that attachment. Changing others to make them be the way you want them to be not only requires an incredible amount of effort and energy, but it doesn't really work, either. Instead of trying to change the other person, it's enough to just let go of your attachment.

There is one thing to keep in mind. I'm telling you to let go of your attachment because it is the problem, but I'm not telling you to forcibly break off the actual relationship with the other person. Once you let go of your attachment, you will be able to deal with the other person comfortably. Then your relationship to that person will flow naturally in whatever direction it goes.

Reflecting on Attachments to People You Dislike

Disliking or resenting someone too much is also an attachment. Becoming uncomfortable and unnatural whenever you deal with the person means that your mind isn't free.

1. Do you have someone you dislike or resent? Who is it? What kind of emotional reaction do you get when you see that person?

2. Was there some event or incident when your feelings of resentment or dislike toward that person began? If so, what was it? Write down what the situation was at the time.

3. Do you have some responsibility for the incident that triggered your dislike? If not, do you think that you have no responsibility at all and that it was the other person's fault? Reflect on the incident carefully, considering whether your words or thoughts might have had even a little effect on what happened.

4. If you were even a little responsible for what happened, it means that you were the victimizer as well as the victim. Have you ever thought that you were at fault?

5. Instead of considering the situation only from your own perspective, try looking at it from the other person's point of view. Try to understand what that person's mindset would have been. If you were also at fault, acknowledge that, close your eyes, bring the other person to mind, and say with sincerity, "I'm sorry. Please forgive me." Write down what you felt through this.

6. Unlike the situation above, you may have been the only one hurt. Even so, look back on the situation again. Consider whether your unconscious thoughts or words affected what happened, even though you weren't aware of it at the time. Try to have an understanding attitude, bearing in mind that the other person may have been in a situation beyond their control, or may have acted that way due to the environment in which they grew up or due to long-established habits. Write down what thoughts come to mind after reflecting on the incident from this perspective.

7. Even if you were the only one hurt, you should let go of victim conscious-ness and hatred, for it will be you and no one else who suffers as long as you hold victim consciousness and hatred in your heart. You can be free only when you release these feelings. Think of it as letting go for your own sake, not for the other person's sake. And make up your mind to have the attitude, "I will no longer suffer with victim consciousness and hatred. I won't resent other people, and I will cultivate my life." Meditate on this, and then write down what you're thinking and feeling.

Reflecting on Attachments to Other Things

People are attached to many things in addition to these three—wealth, power, and people. A tendency toward addiction to things like food, games, alcohol, tobacco, or drugs is also attachment, and psychological conditions such as hypochondria, negative perceptions of the past, anxiety about the future, excessive self-contempt, feelings of superiority, and paranoia are also attachments. What's more, we can say that claiming to be the only one who's right—concluding that only your belief system is right and the rest are wrong—is also a kind of attachment.

You're not free if you lean to one side, whichever side that may be. True freedom can be felt only within harmony and balance. That is the zero-point state, which is not attached to or hung up on anything at all.

Of all the things mentioned above, consider which ones get too much of your attention. Reflect on these and write down how you will recover your balance.

Being Freed from Attachment

The weight of a free soul is zero. But our souls feel heavy and stifled because we've placed so many different burdens on them.

What attachment is burdening and frustrating your soul most now? You could have many different attachments. Write down only the most powerful one.

_____

_____

_____

Do you actually want to let go of that attachment? Or do you just want to hold on to it? What you should let go of is not the object of that attachment but the part of your mind that is the source of the attachment. Examine that part of your mind. Write down what you are feeling.

_____

_____

_____

_____

_____

The question is, do you really want to let go of that attachment? You can let go if you really want to. Do you want to become truly free? Do you really want peace of mind? Reflect on this and write down what you feel.

_____

_____

_____

_____

_____

If you earnestly want to be freed from attachments, read "Meditation for the Freedom of the Soul" on pages 177 to 180 of *I've Decided to Live 120 Years*. Try the meditation, and then write down what you felt.

_____

_____

_____

_____

_____

Let Go of Attachments to Find Peace

Make use of the meditations for letting go of attachments found in the Guided Meditation CD insert of my book *Bird of the Soul*. You can find the book at BestLifeMedia.com.

For one week, try to practice immediately recognizing attachment whenever it's about to arise in your mind. In that moment, instead of concentrating on the object of attachment, try to connect with the feeling of your soul by concentrating on your heart. Correcting the habits of the past requires repeated effort. Write down what you have learned and experienced through such efforts.

Someone whose heart is at peace is blessed. Peace of mind comes when we let go of our attachments. Attachments come from foolishness, and foolishness develops when we don't know the purpose of our lives.

—ILCHI LEE

DON'T FEAR SOLITUDE— ENJOY IT

Read Chapter 8 of *I've Decided to Live 120 Years* before starting this chapter.

I live in that solitude which is painful in youth,
but delicious in the year of maturity.
—ALBERT EINSTEIN

Understanding the Nature of Loneliness

We all come into this world alone and then leave it alone. In between, we meet friends, form families, and belong to communities, connecting and sharing with others. But even in the closest of associations, we suddenly become keenly aware that we are alone. And we end up repeating these questions: Who am I? Where have I come from and where am I going? What is the meaning of my life?

Are you sensitive to loneliness? In what situations do you generally feel a lot of loneliness? What are your emotional states or behavioral patterns at the times when you feel lonely? Examine your condition just as it is and write down what you see.

Where do you think your loneliness comes from? Saying that you're lonely is saying that something is missing, and it's longing for something to fill that lack. What is the concrete reason you feel lonely?

What means do you seek to alleviate your loneliness? There are methods such as meeting people, focusing on work, meditating, exercising, reading, going to movies or watching TV, hiking, playing games, eating, and consuming alcohol. Or you could just wallow in the feeling of loneliness without looking for relief or have trouble finding your way out of it. What do you do when you're lonely? Do the approaches you attempt work well for you?

Do you have any other good ideas for relieving your loneliness? What could you do to make your loneliness disappear?

Have you ever felt lonely even though someone you loved was right beside you? If you have, describe what that feeling was like.

_____

_____

_____

_____

Loneliness felt out of a longing for human affection can be satisfied by the warmth of love. But there is a different, more fundamental loneliness. Everyone experiences moments when the loneliness of existence suddenly digs deep into their heart, even though someone they love is beside them and no matter how much money, power, and popularity they enjoy. The solitude felt in the depths of being is an essential solitude that nothing in this world can resolve.

Go through your memories of when you were young. Didn't you have moments when existential questions came to mind? "Who am I? What is the world? Why do I exist here and now?" These are questions about yourself and the world that you begin to have as your self-awareness grows. If you experienced such questions as you were growing up, describe your memories and feelings from that time.

_____

_____

_____

_____

Did you try to find answers when fundamental questions about your existence came to mind after you had grown up? What did you do, and what did you discover? Or have you given up on finding the answers or forgotten the questions?

No matter how busy we are or how old we may be, the fundamental questions of existence remain in one corner of our hearts until they suddenly and repeatedly come to the surface of our awareness. Have you experienced this? When do you usually feel such solitude?

Why do you think you feel that solitude of being? You search for the reasons and meaning behind it all, and that quest causes you to suffer. What do you think you're trying to find?

The loneliness we feel is a signal flare sent to us by our souls. It's the souls in our hearts waving and impatiently calling us, saying, "I'm here."

The loneliness we feel comes from being cut off from ourselves. No matter how much we try to fill the hole inside us with external things, we cannot help but feel that our hearts are empty shells because our connection with our soul—our true self—has been broken. This is an essential solitude that can never be filled by worldly things. The thirst from that loneliness is quenched only when we recover the connection with our souls.

Entering into Solitude

There is only one way to resolve your essential loneliness, and that is to go deeper and deeper into yourself—until you discover your soul, your true self, your true nature, and until you experience oneness with the fundamental life of the cosmos. You can find answers to your fundamental questions only through inner searching and reflection.

It's all right to be lonely. It's okay to find yourself alone. In fact, you should actively seek loneliness and solitude. Do you think being lonely and alone is bad? It isn't. Taking time for solitude means you are immersed in the search for your being. Countless philosophers and artists who have come and gone from this world, including saints such as the Buddha and Jesus, have spent long hours in solitude. They attempted constant inner exploration with an earnest desire to face their own true nature and discover the meaning of existence.

Everyone needs times like those. Enter into solitude completely. Don't refuse it. Only then can you encounter your true self, your soul. Go within yourself, as if questing for inner treasure. Discover what riches await you there.

Try the following meditative practice for experiencing brilliant solitude. Take time alone in nature, and find a secluded space where you can focus entirely on yourself without being disturbed by others. Sitting in a meditative posture, straighten your back and close your eyes. Slowly get your breathing under control. When your mind is calm and tranquil, open your inner eyes and look into the soul in your heart. Meditate, asking yourself the following questions one by one.

Who am I, really?

Am I my body? Am I my emotions? Am I my thoughts? If I'm not these things, what is my true self, and where is it? Am I feeling my true self right now? Find who you really are.

How much have I been separated from my true self?

The more genuine your feelings of separation from your true self, the more quickly you can recover your connection with it.

What does my soul earnestly want?

Try to feel your body as you keep breathing. Continuing, try to feel the energy of your soul in your heart. Feel what it is your soul energy earnestly wants.

What the soul energy in your heart earnestly desires is unity with divinity, becoming Shinmyung, a brightening of shin energy in your brain. Do the Jungchoong, Kijang, Shinmyung energy meditation described on pages 65 and 66 in this workbook. After feeling the energy between the palms of your hands, send the energy coming from your palms into your abdomen, chest, face, and brain, in that order.

When you've completed the final stage, Shinmyung training, lower your hands and place them over your knees. Concentrate your mind on the crown of your head and then imagine bright, numinous energy descending into your body from there. Feel each and every one of your cells vibrating as the energy reaches them. You're receiving the energy of the cosmos, the love and blessings of the divine. Human and divine meeting as one is the moment of divine-human unity, the instant when brilliant solitude shines.

Am I really alone?

Are you alone right now? Try to feel what is with you now. The life energy of the cosmos is completely filling each of the cells throughout your body. You are encountering the fundamental life energy of the cosmos, which has existed from the beginning. You are alone but not alone, for cosmic life energy fills you. Your divine nature, which is connected and one with the entire universe, is shining. You're in brilliant solitude.

Write down what you felt through this meditation.

_____

_____

_____

_____

_____

_____

_____

_____

_____

_____

_____

Did you feel brilliant solitude through this meditation? Those who are familiar with meditation can get a deep feeling, but beginners may not. It's great even if you only got a tiny feeling for it. All you have to do is continue developing the seed of that sense. It will lead you to feel that the moments you spend encountering your true self are really a time of truth and fullness.

For doing meditation well, you need to develop your ki energy sense. You're not just concentrating dryly with thought alone; energy phenomena are amplified when you go with the flow of ki energy. This is because both the soul and divinity are energy phenomena arising in your consciousness and in your body.

Enjoying Brilliant Solitude

Brilliant solitude and ordinary solitude are different. Ordinary solitude is just being alone. Brilliant solitude, however, is being alone but not alone. It's a fullness that comes in the moment when, alone, you connect with everything as one.

When you look at the stars in the night sky, when you walk on a quiet path through the woods, when you watch the setting sun, when you meditate and practice alone—these moments come to you when you're alone yet connected with all things. These are the moments when you taste brilliant solitude. This is when you realize that the fundamental loneliness within you can never be filled by another person or by anything outside you, that this lonely emptiness is only filled by being completely one with the great life force of the universe.

So when you're alone, enjoy the solitude. Take time when you're completely by yourself to shut down all the noisy thoughts and emotions, the voices screeching in your head, and enter into solitude, burrowing deep within. Do it until your soul awakens and you encounter the divinity of the cosmos, until you feel the self that is one with all things in the infinite love and blessings of divinity.

I compare people who embrace brilliant solitude to spines. Try doing the following spine meditation:

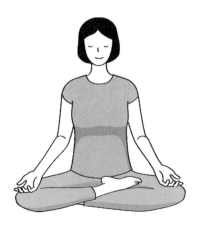

Sit in a meditative posture and straighten your lower back. Gently close your eyes and place your hands comfortably over your knees, palms facing up. Starting in your tailbone, straighten and align your lumbar, thoracic, and cervical vertebrae. Fully open the energy point in the crown of your head, and imagine the pure, clear energy of the universe coming down into your head. Visualize that energy descending from your head along your spine into your tailbone and then spreading throughout your entire body.

Try to feel your spine maintaining your body's center and balance. Your spine supports Heaven above and connects to the earth below. Your whole body will feel comfortable only if your spine is centered exactly.

In that state, try to feel your organs, legs, and head. Does your body feel comfortable overall?

Now, tilting your upper body about 30 degrees to the left, try to lean into your left hip and lower back. Keep holding that posture. Does your body feel uncomfortable? How would the organs, muscles, and other parts of your body change if you held that posture for a long time? What things would happen in your body and mind?

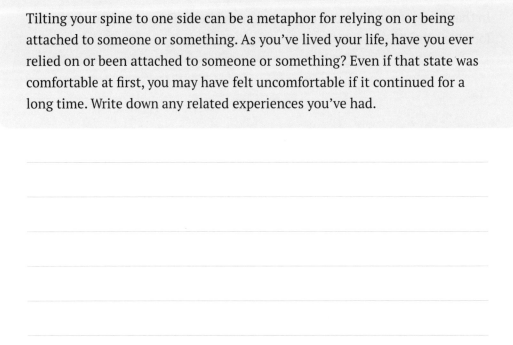

Tilting your spine to one side can be a metaphor for relying on or being attached to someone or something. As you've lived your life, have you ever relied on or been attached to someone or something? Even if that state was comfortable at first, you may have felt uncomfortable if it continued for a long time. Write down any related experiences you've had.

Those who would complete their souls in brilliant solitude must think of their upright spines. When you are leaning to one side and relying on or stuck in something, you cannot feel the whole. You feel the whole when you are completely alone and lonely. When the loneliness of being reaches deep into your heart, a bright light breaks out of the darkness. Then great solitude changes into brilliant light.

Telling you to live like a backbone does not mean you should discontinue interactions with people and be alone all the time. It means you should find your definite center. That center is the soul, your true self. Deal with people, or the world, centered on the feeling of your soul like a well-balanced body centered on its spine. Instead of being led about by other people or by the world, stand on your own two feet, centered in your soul. That is true self-reliance.

When you are able to be self-reliant, you're finally ready to truly love. Instead of just trying to rely on or get love from other people, you become able to share the energy of pure love pouring from the soul—your center—without hoping for reward. That is a peace and love for all. The wisdom and power to bring harmony to the world emerges when you can look at the world with this awareness.

Do you want to realize a life of self-reliance with a spine-like center? Think about how you will apply this idea in your relationships, personal activities, and social activities, and write down your thoughts below.

Relationships

Who: _____

How: _____

_____

Who: _____

How: _____

_____

Personal Activities

What Activities: _____

How: _____

_____

What Activities: _____

How: _____

_____

Social Activities

What Activities: _____

How: _____

_____

What Activities: _____

How: _____

_____

Write down what changes you experienced after a week of acting on the plan you made above.

_____

_____

_____

_____

_____

If you go forward with brilliant solitude in your heart, you become what I call a truly fragrant person, one who has the greatest possible attractiveness.
—ILCHI LEE

GIVE YOUR BRAIN HOPES AND DREAMS

Read Chapter 9 of *I've Decided to Live 120 Years* before starting this chapter.

Years may wrinkle the skin, but to give up enthusiasm wrinkles the soul.
—SAMUEL ULLMAN

Checking Your Thoughts on Aging

At this point in your journey, how do you think about aging? Do you think about it positively or negatively?

Use your thoughts to complete the sentence below. Write down what thoughts and feelings you currently have about older people.

Older people are

_____

_____

_____

_____

Do you think of yourself as younger or older than your actual age? What is your reason for thinking that way?

_____

_____

_____

_____

According to one study led by Professor Andrew Steptoe of University College London, people who thought of themselves as younger than their actual age lived approximately 50 percent more years during the course of the study than those who thought of themselves as older than they are. Ultimately, the functioning of our bodies and minds changes according to the information in our brains.

What information are you giving your brain, and what external information are you accepting concerning your old age?

Boldly reject socially accepted ideas that don't help you live your later years in health, happiness, and fullness. Give your brain positive information.

Close your eyes, then picture yourself healthy and full of energy in your later years. Write down what you pictured and how you felt.

If you have thought about aging negatively, try to correct your information about older people and use a positive idea to complete the sentence below. Close your eyes again, then repeat the affirmation you created to yourself. Write down what you felt.

Older people are

What you felt:

Providing Your Brain with Vitamin H

Managing your brain means managing your body and mind. Look at your lifestyle again to see how you're caring for your brain health. For each of the following categories, choose Good, Fair, or Poor. Write down what you're doing now, your current condition, and what you need to improve in the future.

Lifestyle	Evaluation	Current Efforts and Condition	Areas to Improve
Plenty of Rest and Sleep	Good Fair Poor		
Regular Exercise	Good Fair Poor		
Balanced Meals	Good Fair Poor		
Appropriate Social Activities	Good Fair Poor		
Good Personal Relationships	Good Fair Poor		

I've Decided to Live 120 Years Personal Workbook

The lifestyle areas listed on the previous page are the most fundamental elements for maintaining good brain health. But in addition to these, there is another method that activates the brain most powerfully. That method is to have hopes and dreams in which the brain can immerse itself; in other words, it's having a purpose.

People who had a goal in life were found to have a risk of death 15 percent lower than those who did not. Having a specific purpose in life means having hopes and dreams about the future.

Hope is vitamin H, which instills our brains with vitality. I'm in the habit of explaining this by calling brains with a vitamin H deficiency "Dark Brains" and brains with plenty of vitamin H "Power Brains."

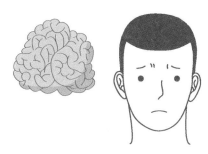 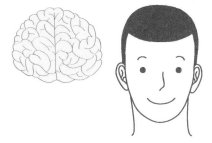

Dark Brain	Power Brain
• Status Quo/Regression	• Growth/Development Oriented
• Emits Weak Energy	• Emits Lively Energy
• Negative Mindset	• Positive Mindset
• Worries and Fears	• Passion and Courage
• Disinterest	• Interest/Curiosity
• Reduced/Lost Ambition	• Full of Ambition
• Nonproductive	• Productive
• Habitual/Inert	• Creative
• Anxious	• Peaceful

As you look at the two images and descriptions on the previous page, try to feel and compare the conditions of each kind of brain. What feelings do you get, and what differences do you sense?

_____

_____

_____

Which of the two types above is your brain presently closest to? Why do you feel that way?

_____

_____

_____

If your brain's condition is close to the Dark Brain, then it's important that you first acknowledge that the responsibility for making your brain this way lies with you. Reflect on and write down the habits you've had in managing your brain.

_____

_____

_____

If your brain's condition is close to the Power Brain, write down your positive habits and how you've been providing your brain with vitamin H.

_____

_____

_____

_____

Do you worry that your brain is a Dark Brain? If so, then immediately stop worrying about it! Worry is a thought pattern of the Dark Brain. Instead, get out of habits of inertia right away.

Here's some hopeful news for you: our brains have amazing resiliency and plasticity. Not only do new neurons develop even when we're older, but new networks are created between neurons, and brain function can improve. No matter how old you may be, you can experience and challenge yourself with new things, changing and stimulating your brain.

LIVING A PURPOSEFUL LIFE

Look back on how you lived your life today. Did you live it habitually without much of a plan or much change? Or did you carry out a plan for the day and live it productively and creatively?

_____

_____

_____

_____

Today, did you let your brain be, allowing Dark Brain thought patterns to operate? Or did you strive to become a Power Brain? Recall your brain condition and write down the attitude you had in dealing with your brain and with your life.

What about your lifestyle patterns? Do you tend to continuously repeat the familiar without much change? Or do you make changes and challenge yourself, even if only in small ways? Thinking back on the previous week or month, analyze your lifestyle patterns. Write down how you changed and how you challenged yourself.

Changes and challenges don't just mean doing very novel, consequential things. It's about living a purposeful life. Something "purposeful" could be the great purpose of your life, or it could be a short-term goal.

If you have a precise purpose or goal, then in order to achieve it you can't help but first engage in self-renewal. You set up and prepare a schedule and plan, and you allocate time for taking care of your physical condition, for managing your mind, and for nurturing your personal relationships. Otherwise you'll get no new ideas or energy, and despite your resolution, you could easily give up and burn out within a few days.

What purpose and goals do you have for tomorrow, and what do you plan to do? Set up a plan for tomorrow. Also set aside plenty of time for self-renewal such as taking care of your body, mind, and spirit.

Time	What to Do	Check/Reflect

Think about the state of your brain as you carried out your plan for the day. Was it closer to a Dark Brain or a Power Brain?

Did a day spent planning and focusing on achieving a purpose feel different from a day lived with no purpose or plan in mind? Write down what you felt.

The areas of "superager" brains that are activated more than those of ordinary seniors are the areas where we handle emotion or sentiment, not those involved with cognition or thinking. These areas are activated when we keep doing difficult tasks, whether mental or physical.

A high level of activity in these areas of the brain causes us to feel negative emotions such as tiredness and frustration. These are the feelings we get when we wrestle with a difficult math problem or push ourselves to our physical limits during exercise. You may develop uncomfortable weariness of body and mind when you have to focus intensely mentally, but you can develop your mental muscles to give yourself a sharper memory and more powerful focus.

I've Decided to Live 120 Years Personal Workbook

Just living comfortably and easily without any particular purpose, goal, or plan is not the best course to follow for brain health. Your brain is activated when you carry out a plan to achieve a goal that you've set. The hopes and dreams given to your brain by purpose and goals are vitamin H. So establish a purpose and goal your brain can focus on. The higher your purpose, the better your brain will focus.

What is your purpose/goal? If it's not clear yet, think carefully and decide.

Short-Term Purpose/Goal (for example, one month):

_____

_____

_____

_____

Long-Term Purpose/Goal (for example, one year or longer):

_____

_____

_____

_____

_____

How are you preparing and renewing yourself to achieve your purpose? What parts of yourself do you feel need to be improved, and how will you improve them?

A basic principle of the brain's operation is that it improves when stimulated and declines without stimulation. Seniors can no longer use age as an excuse, claiming that a rusty brain keeps them from doing or learning something new. Our brains are able to learn until the final moments of our lives.

Think about and write down new things you want to attempt, challenges you want to take up, and things you want to learn.

BRAIN MEDITATION FOR POSITIVE ENERGY

Now try experiencing positive affirmation, consciously choosing repeating thoughts that will have a positive impact on your future. First you have to decide on the message.

Think about what message could give you strength and hope. It might be the mission statement you wrote on page 57, or it might be an ideal picture of yourself in the future. Create one or two sentences as a positive affirmation to give to yourself. Try to write the message you are most in need of right now, in your present situation; you can always revise it in the future.

Try doing Brain Meditation for Positive Energy, based on the contents of pages 208 to 211 of *I've Decided to Live 120 Years*. Afterwards write or draw a picture of what you felt.

If you repeatedly practice this meditation in your daily life, it will provide your brain with positive energy and help you become a creative, peaceful Power Brain.

Asking ourselves who we really are, searching for an answer to that question, and becoming our true selves—this is really our greatest task in life and the greatest motivation we can give our brains.

—ILCHI LEE

CULTIVATE YOURSELF CONTINUOUSLY

Read Chapter 10 of *I've Decided to Live 120 Years* before starting this chapter.

Just as a candle cannot burn without fire,
men cannot live without a spiritual life.
—BUDDHA

Understanding Three Realizations About Life

Our lives might be defined as a "school for enlightenment." All the things you have seen, heard, and experienced since you were born into this world are precious assets you have accumulated. Piece by piece, you have been learning the meaning of life contained in all those moments, whether they were happy, sad, or painful.

The second half of life is a time when you lay out all those fragments and fit them together one way or another as you meditate on their true meaning. You do this to complete the profound and mysterious puzzle of the life that has been given to you.

There are three great realizations you will encounter as you put together the puzzle of life. The first is this: **Life is suffering**.

What kinds of things have troubled you and caused you to suffer in your life so far? Write down everything you can think of as you take a long look back over your life.

Have you had moments of keen awareness when you realized, "Oh, life is really painful"? If so, describe your experience and feelings at such times.

When you became acutely aware of life's suffering, what did you learn through that realization? Did those experiences and lessons affect your attitudes in dealing with people and with life itself?

Our study of life really begins when we start realizing that life is suffering, for we come to reflect more on the meaning of life when we have hardship than when we're joyful. "Why live such a difficult, painful life? What does it all mean?" Have you had times when you thought this way?

Those moments when we feel the suffering of life are agonizing. But when we overcome that pain and, as time passes, look at how our lives have unfolded, we realize that rapid inner growth—including patience, tolerance, courage, and the strength to never give up—were made possible through that suffering. As the saying goes, "No pain, no gain." In the same way, we might say, "No pain, no growth." If we deal with the world out of gratitude for the bitter suffering of life, it actually becomes a pain that benefits us.

Life is impermanent. This is the second great realization in life. "Impermanence" also signifies that life is pointless and meaningless, but its fundamental meaning is that there is nothing that doesn't change. The principle of all things in nature is that everything is always changing; nothing remains in the same state. Nature changes, people change, you change, and the world changes.

Have you ever felt that life is impermanent? Have you felt the pointlessness and suffering of life as you watched some situation or thing changing, something you had hoped wouldn't change? Write down any experience you have had with this.

It's not only other people and external things that change. You, too, have been changing continuously. Your body has been changing, and your mind has been changing. Reflect on how your body and mind have been changing. How you felt yesterday was different from how you feel today. Who knows how it may change tomorrow? Reflect on the principle of impermanence ceaselessly arising inside you, and write down what you feel.

What do you feel when an object or situation you'd hoped wouldn't change does change, and when you watch your body—which once seemed like it would be young forever—declining, little by little?

Maybe you should compare the changes in yourself so far with the changes you'll experience as you pass on to old age and death. Suppose that you're older and are facing death. When you realize that you can take nothing with you—not the wealth you have acquired in this world, not your beautiful clothes and accessories, not even a single hair on your head—how will you feel then? Imagine the emptiness and remorse you will feel about how you've struggled so much—and for what? Write down your thoughts.

One of the main reasons we feel that life is suffering is that we don't readily accept the truth of impermanence. We hope that the happiness we feel and our environment won't change, we hope the person we love won't have a change of heart, and we hope our youth and vigor will last. But waves of suffering rush over us every time we see change in the things we hoped would never change.

The strength to swim out of those waves of suffering begins in just accepting the basic fact of impermanence. If there is anything in this world that doesn't change, it is the very truth that there is nothing that doesn't change. When we tranquilly accept this second truth of life—impermanence—we can go on to the next stage. This is the stage where we can actually enjoy the waves of life instead of being swept away by them.

What is this stage? It's a way of emerging from suffering and impermanence to enjoy the waves of life! It's awakening to **nothingness**—or **muah** in Korean (literally "no-self" or "egolessness"). This is the third great realization of life. It speaks of the self that has awakened to oneness with all things.

Awakening to muah could be an endlessly difficult problem if you think of it as being difficult, or it could be incredibly simple if you think of it as easy.

There is a gate you have to pass through in order to go on to the stage of muah. Check your perspective through the following questions.

We have a visible body and an invisible spirit. Which of these do you think is your essence? Why do you think that way?

Are you living a life centered in the body or a life centered in the spirit? On which of these do you place more importance? If you were to express this as a ratio of body to spirit, what would it be?

You can't experience muah through a life that places importance only on the body—or, more precisely put, on the desires and emotions that come from the body. Muah is a state you can feel only when you've transcended your small self, your ego. When viewed with egocentric eyes, "self" and "other" appear different, and all things seem separated from each other. When viewed with the eyes of muah, though, the self is one with all things, and one with the universe.

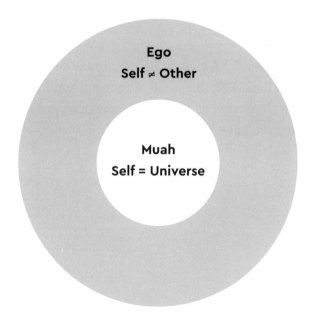

You must open your eyes to another world that exists behind the visible body and material world: the invisible world of energy. That energy is our essence and the substance of all things in the cosmos. Energy is the source of all things in creation, from invisible spirit to visible matter, and is creation itself.

Realizing that energy is your substance, and that this energy transcends your small self and is interconnected with the life energy of the cosmos—that is the enlightenment of nothingness, muah. It's awakening not to the little self, but to the great self that is one with the universe.

As you've lived your life, have you ever had the feeling that you'd transcended your small self and were connected with the whole, with nature or the cosmos? If so, when was it? Describe what it felt like.

Repeat the meditation for feeling brilliant solitude described in this workbook on pages 191 and 192, Chapter 8. After transcending your small self and connecting with the energy of divinity, the life energy of the cosmos, write down the feeling you have.

I coined the term "LifeParticles" as another expression for energy. I created this term by adding the meaning of life energy to the concept of the elementary particle, the smallest unit of matter revealed by science so far. Our bodies and minds are made up of energy—in other words, LifeParticles—and in fact everything in the universe is made up of LifeParticles. I created an image of the source from which the life energy of the cosmos is emitted, which I call the LifeParticle Sun, and I have been teaching people a method of energy meditation for receiving LifeParticles from that sun and being one with life energy.

If you want do know how to do a meditation using LifeParticles, find a LifeParticle Energy Meditation video online at ChangeYourEnergy.com or a CD or my book *LifeParticle Meditation* at BestLifeMedia.com. This will help you get the feeling of being one with cosmic life energy and experiencing muah.

Understanding Three Elements of a Spiritual Life

Do you want to finish your life after just living any old way with the awareness that life is suffering and impermanent? Or do you want to end your life after realizing that your substance is one with the infinite life energy of the cosmos, and then living for peace and completion? Write down your thoughts.

To put the question another way, do you want to be free from life's yoke of suffering and anguish, or do you just want to continue living that life of bondage?

Anyone who's human wants to be free. We want to be happy. We want to be at peace. What we're saying, though, is that the true freedom, happiness, and peace we want is not found in a life centered only on the body. Let's definitely recognize this fact, for confinement, unhappiness, and anguish exist in a life centered on the body. True freedom, happiness, and peace is possible through a life centered in the soul. That is a spiritual life, a life for the growth and completion of the soul.

Of course, since we have bodies, we shouldn't ignore their needs. But instead of being led about by the desires and emotions of the body, a spiritual life is one in which we master them, managing our bodies and feelings. We manage and use our bodies and life energy as tools for the growth and completion of our souls, which is the top priority of our lives. This is about clearly understanding something essential: the soul is our purpose, and the body is a means for realizing that purpose.

Do you feel the need to eliminate or add some things in your current life for the growth and completion of your soul? Select three elements for each of these, and write down your reasons as well.

Elements That Should Be Eliminated

For example: How I lash out at people when I'm stressed.

1. _____

2. _____

3. _____

Elements That Should Be Added

For example: Having more patience and tolerance for myself and others.

1. _____

2. _____

3. _____

I propose three concrete elements for living a spiritual life, which you can see in the diagram below. The first is sustained self-cultivation, the second is Hongik—the sharing and giving of benevolence—and the third is being close to nature. A combination of these three is perfect for the completion of the soul; they come together to form a whole life.

In this chapter, let's study self-cultivation.

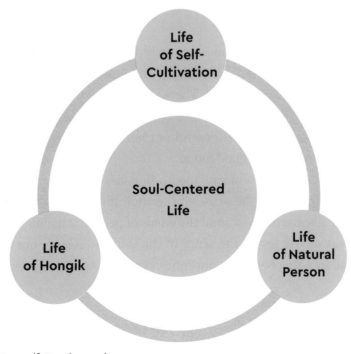

Adding Meditation to Daily Life

Meditation is a daily practice I really want to recommend for cultivating your-self continuously.

Have you been meditating? If you have, what effects have you been able to achieve through meditation? Write down the effects you've experienced through meditation, whether they are physical, mental, or spiritual.

Many studies have shown that meditation reduces stress, stabilizes the mind, and creates positive emotions. When you meditate, your brain waves reach an alpha-wave or theta-wave level. There's a decrease in the secretion of hor-mones such as cortisol and adrenaline, which are released in stressful situ-ations, and an increase in the secretion of hormones such as serotonin and oxytocin, which put us in a good mood.

The main reason I recommend meditation, besides these various positive effects, is to avoid losing the sense of the soul. It's easy to lose the sense of the soul as we live hectic lives amid the chaos of packed schedules and surging emotions. But we can revive the sense of the soul and restore our connection with the soul by going back into our inner world through meditation.

Experience "Breathing Meditation for Encountering the Soul," introduced on pages 224 and 225 of *I've Decided to Live 120 Years*, and then write down what you felt while doing it. Did you feel your soul and experience a connection with your soul?

Another effect you can get through meditation, from the perspective of the spiritual life, is to experience being one with the life energy of the cosmos. There are limits to the depth of that experience with just one attempt, though. It is true that a great deal of effort and practice are required.

I introduced a method on pages 226 to 228 of *I've Decided to Live 120 Years* for briefly experiencing that. Write down what you felt after practicing "Meditation for Being One with the Life Energy of the Cosmos."

Continuing the practice for a long time while in one fixed meditative posture is not the only way to meditate. Nothing is set in stone that says you have to do meditation a certain way. Experiencing substantial effects is more important than form. If thoughts and feelings keep arising in your head no matter how long you sit in a meditative posture, then it's actually better to get up and try meditating in another form. Whatever lets you shake off the endless thread of tangled thoughts, stimulating stable, peaceful, positive energy in your mind, that is meditation.

Meditation and living are not separate things; life becomes meditation, and meditation becomes life. This is why I consider meditation in daily life important. Try adding the following meditation practices to your daily routine.

Breathing Meditation

"Breathing Meditation for Encountering the Soul," mentioned earlier, is a good example. Feel your life energy and soul as you meditate, going with the rhythm as you breathe in and out.

Walking Meditation

Walk counting your steps as you match them to your breathing. For example, inhale while you take four steps and exhale while you take another four steps. Adjust the number of steps to the length of your breaths.

Nature Meditation

Charge up on life energy as you commune with nature—the sunlight, trees, sounds of rushing water, bird songs, and flowers.

Tea Meditation

Feel calmness and tranquility of mind as you smell the aroma of tea, slowly savor its flavor, and feel its warmth spreading through your body.

Resting Meditation

Resting is also a good form of meditation. While lying down or comfortably leaning against the back of a chair, slowly relax your body. Look within and charge yourself with life energy as you breathe.

Evening Meditation in Bed

Breathe very slowly as you lie in bed. It's okay to do a count, if you wish. For example, inhale while counting to five and then exhale while counting to five again. Increase this number according to the length of your breath. If you drift off when your breathing is deep, you can enjoy a good night's sleep and be charged up with life energy.

Energy Training Meditation

You can meditate while doing certain movements or holding postures, as in yoga, tai chi, and qigong. Your brain waves will stabilize, and your body and mind will grow calm as your energy and blood circulation are stimulated by the practice.

Apply one of these lifestyle meditation practices each day for one week, and then write down what you felt while doing it.

Day	Meditation	What You Felt
Day 1		
Day 2		
Day 3		
Day 4		
Day 5		
Day 6		
Day 7		

Continuing Self-Development

You need self-development and self-discipline in the process of making yourself a better person. You might have pursued self-development during your period of success for the purpose of improving your résumé. During retirement, however, you can engage in self-cultivation for the pure joy and inner satisfaction that comes from working to make yourself better, for maturity of character and completion of the soul.

It's about forming an ideal self-image—the person you dream of becoming, "I will be this kind of human being"—and then making choices and acting in ways that let you reach that self-image.

Considered a role model for self-development, U.S. founding father Benjamin Franklin at the age of 20 made it his life's goal to develop his character. He decided on 13 virtues and strove to practice them. These are the virtues he targeted: temperance, silence, order, resolution, frugality, industry, sincerity, justice, moderation, cleanliness, tranquility, chastity, and humility.

What is your own ideal self-image? Close your eyes and picture the kind of character you want to have as a person.

In a single sentence, write what virtues you want to develop to realize your self-image, and what those virtues mean concretely.

Do you consider your self-image to be feasible to achieve or just an idealistic dream that is out of your reach?

If you consider your self-image possible, then you will definitely be able to achieve it. Even if you think it's an idealistic dream, you shouldn't stop striving to make it come true. What's important is how diligently you work to reach it and how you grow through each and every part of that process. That is the beauty of self-development.

As long as we live, we should realize our creative nature through unending self-cultivation. We should work to renew ourselves every day until that final moment when our hearts and brains stop working. Today should somehow be different from yesterday, and tomorrow should be better than today.

What specific steps will you take to reach your desired self-image? Write down things to act on in your daily life.

Act on the plan you have made for one week, and then write down what you are feeling.

If we compete with anyone, it is with the person we were yesterday.
—ILCHI LEE

SHARE AND GIVE

Read Chapter 11 of *I've Decided to Live 120 Years* before starting this chapter.

It's not how much we give but how much love we put into giving.
—MOTHER TERESA

Checking Your Soul's Satisfaction

The greatest regret people express when facing death is that they lacked the courage to live lives true to themselves. The entity that seeks to live an authentic life is not your thoughts, desires, or emotions. It is your true self—your soul.

We feel that life is hard when the energy of our souls has shrunk and stagnated. Our souls don't want their energy fields to be trapped inside us. They want to expand widely and freely. We want to express our soul energy through creative, meaningful activities, through sharing and interacting with others. Then we feel, "Oh, I'm living the life my heart truly wants!"

We can check how much we're causing our souls to grow at any time, not just in the final moments before we die. We can look back on our lives and ask our hearts this question: "If I were to die right now, am I confident that I wouldn't regret my life?"

Close your eyes and focus all your senses inward. Try to feel your chest. That's where the energy of your soul is. As you feel that energy, reflect on the life you've lived. Then ask yourself, "If I die right now, in this moment, am I confident that I won't regret my life?"

Write down the reaction you feel in your chest, just as it is.

_____

_____

_____

_____

Close your eyes and feel your chest. How satisfied do you feel with your life? What percentage of your heart do you feel has been filled with the energy of your soul? Get a feel for how full—what percentage—you want it to be when you meet death. Use lines or color to fill in the following circles—the left circle for the satisfaction of your soul now, the right circle for the satisfaction you hope your soul will feel before you die.

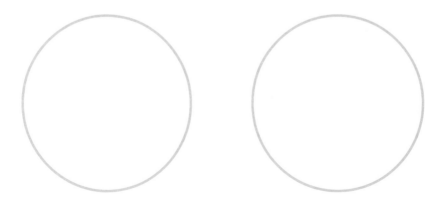

Current Satisfaction (   )%   Desired Satisfaction before Death (   )%

Close your eyes again and reflect on what you regret about your life. You might regret something you've done wrong or something you've failed to achieve. Try to sense why your heart isn't completely full. After taking plenty of time to meditate, write down what you felt.

Regrets About What You've Done Wrong

1. _____

_____

2. _____

_____

3. _____

_____

Regrets About What You've Failed to Achieve

1. _____

_____

2. _____

_____

3. _____

_____

Reasons Why Your Heart Isn't Completely Full

1. _____

_____

2. _____

_____

3. _____

_____

Given the opportunity to live out your remaining years, how do you want to live? How do you want to resolve each of the regrets you have about your life? You still have a chance—a chance to create a life without regrets, a chance to meet death without regret. Think carefully about how you will resolve each of the issues involved in your current regrets, and then write down your solutions. Some things cannot be resolved in person, for instance, when they involve a person who has passed away. When you have remorse toward someone no longer in your life, close your eyes, bring the person to mind, and have a true conversation with them in the world of consciousness. Through this practice, release all the emotional energy you have been carrying. Applying the lessons you learned from them to your future is also important.

How to Resolve Your Regrets About What You've Done Wrong

1. _____

_____

2. _____

_____

3. _____

_____

How to Resolve Your Regrets About What You've Failed to Achieve

1. _____

_____

2. _____

_____

3. _____

_____

How to Resolve the Reasons Why Your Heart Isn't Completely Full

1. _____

_____

2. _____

_____

3. _____

Identifying What Your Soul Wants

Looking back on your life with regret means that you have failed to satisfy your soul in what it truly wants. What is it, then, that your soul wants? To live a satisfying life, first of all, you have to identify what that is.

What our souls truly want, that is the soul's purpose. What is that purpose? To what end does the soul seek to grow and develop?

The soul wants to grow brighter, to expand, and to be more complete. Ultimately, it dreams of unity with the divine, the life energy of the cosmos. That is the dream of being one with Heaven and returning to the original Source of life. Our souls do not want to cower in darkness. They want to lift their bright faces and grow toward the dream of completion like sunflowers looking toward the sun.

How, then, can we make the soul's energy grow?

The law by which our souls grow is simple. It is this: The energy of the soul grows greater the more it's shared.

The energy system of the middle dahnjon, or heart chakra, in our chests operates in a peculiar way. It functions in a way that is the exact opposite of a bank account in which money that is saved and not used grows with interest. The energy of the soul, in contrast, fills the heart to the extent that it is shared and used. It's an amazing kind of account, with a balance that actually decreases the less it is shared and used.

Sharing is a way to increase the account of the soul. This is Hongik, working widely for the good of others and the world. The soul grows and is completed through Hongik.

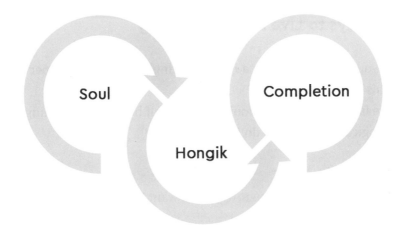

The soul completes its journey through acts that benefit others (Hongik).

As you've lived your life, have you experienced the law that says the energy of the soul grows greater the more it's shared? Have you ever felt a kind of fullness and satisfaction in your heart when you've shared what you have, even if it's in a very small way, or have helped another person? If you have experienced this, write down what happened. How did your heart feel then?

What you felt was the joy and happiness of the soul. This is different from the joy you feel when your desires or greed are satisfied. This is a pure joy, one that is unconditional and doesn't look for reward. When this joy is growing, it means that the energy of the soul is growing.

Finding Ways to Live a Life of Sharing

How can you practice Hongik, a life of sharing? Are there any specific methods for this?

There is something you should ask yourself before approaching this on a methodological level: "What do I want to share?"

Write down your thoughts about what you want to share.

_____

_____

_____

_____

_____

_____

When we think of "sharing," things like material contributions or volunteer activities commonly come to mind. What's important, though, is not the action seen on the outside. It's the attitude you put into the action. What we truly want to share and what we *should* share is our hearts, the energy of our souls. The energy of the soul can be called "love," but to put it more precisely, it is the mind that wants to help people, a heart of Hongik. Regardless of the form your sharing takes, first check whether you have this heart.

Do you want to be of help to people? Feel your heart if you are willing to share your heart energy. Write down what you feel.

If your heart is ready, let's think hard about the next methodological level. What you need to identify before deciding how you want to share is "What can I share?" Sharing means giving of the things you have. First identify what it is you have. Then all you need to do later is decide which of those things you want to share.

What you have isn't limited to material things visible to the eye. You also have talents, time, a soul, and spirit. The experience, knowledge, skills, and beliefs you've been accumulating, even your time—all of these are unseen things you can share.

Write down in detail what it is you can share.

You might think you don't have that much to share. If that is the case, here are some suggestions of things you may be able to share.

Contributing Materially

1. **Monetary Contributions**

   Of the many ways to share, one of the simplest is donating money. Think carefully about what individuals or organizations will receive your donation and for what purpose it will be used.

2. **Material Donations**

   Material goods (works of art, accessories, clothing, etc.) can also be shared. Especially as we get older, it occurs to us that these are things we have to let go of before we die, anyway. It's a good idea to simplify your life as you put your affairs in order instead of continuing to pile up things that you don't absolutely need. You'll be able to feel the joy of sharing while you live if you give these things to your family, friends, and the needy.

3. **Participation in Organizations**

   You can also contribute by creating, running, or taking part in the activities of an organization whose purpose is to make the world a better place—for example, an organization set up to serve the vulnerable or provide jobs. Such organizations can take a variety of forms, from non-profit or social corporations to for-profit businesses donating profits to a cause that's important to you.

Contributing with Talent

1. **Activities for Sharing Talent**

   There are many ways in which you can share and teach the skills and experience you have. For example, you could give lectures or provide consultation in artistic fields such as playing musical instruments, drawing, writing, and crafts; in technical fields necessary in modern daily life; or in fields of knowledge such as finances, the humanities, and languages. Another good method is teaching mind-body health practices you know, such as yoga or qigong, or even simple methods like those in this book, including One-Minute Exercise, Longevity Walking, and Belly Button Healing. You could participate in a club or provide your services at a cultural center, shelter, senior center, or similar facility.

2. **Creative Activities Using Talent**

   Although you can share and teach your talents, meeting people directly as I just suggested, you can also share through the creative activities you engage in personally. For example, if you are skilled in music, art, or writing, you could express your inspirations or messages through your creations. By doing so, you could inspire the people who come across your work to live for the growth and completion of their souls and to contribute to making the world a better place.

Contributing with Time

Those who think that they don't have special talents or skills can actively take part in a variety of volunteer activities in their communities, if they make the time to do so. Through such activities, you can taste the joy of using the time you've been given in meaningful, rewarding ways.

Sharing Online

By using online resources such as blogs and social media to express your feelings and convey a message, you could inspire other people, leading them to take part in creating a culture of more open, caring interaction.

Sharing in Daily Life

You can practice sharing in your daily life as well as in special activities. Smile and greet those you meet more cheerfully. Express joy, gratitude, and love more often. You can teach simple health practices, and you can listen sincerely to the worries of another person. You can turn your daily life itself into an opportunity to practice sharing.

After reading all these suggestions, think once more about what you can share, and write down your thoughts.

_____

_____

_____

_____

_____

_____

_____

_____

Have you realized that there is a lot you have and a lot you can share? Everything you've seen, heard, felt, and obtained in this world can be shared. And the energy of your soul, and your love, grows when you share all these things without holding back. The more you share, the fuller your heart grows.

When there is nothing left to grasp at, when you've given and shared it all, when you've loved fully so your heart is filled with joy and satisfaction, then in the moment you die you will have no remorse. And feeling that "I now have no regrets in my life," you will be able to close your eyes in peace and blessedness.

Planning for a Life of Sharing After Retirement

After you retire, you can embody a life of sharing because you have more freedom in many ways. You can also greatly expand your sharing, going beyond your family and friends to your neighbors and community.

Close your eyes and picture what you can share and want to share in old age. Set up a detailed plan for how you will practice a life of sharing in order to live without regrets.

Target of Sharing	Things I Have That I Can and Want to Share	Detailed Sharing/ Activity Plan
Family		
Friends/ Acquaintances		
Neighbors/ Community		

Beginning a Life of Sharing Now

You don't have to wait until you retire to live a life of sharing. You can start right now, whatever your age. The joy of sharing is felt immediately when you act. Don't put off tasting joy until sometime in the distant future. If you want to feel the joy and happiness of the soul in your present life, practice sharing right now.

Sharing with People Who Are Close

Of the people close to you, think about whom you will share with first. Then find out what it is that person needs. Hongik isn't a unilateral love that just gives what we want to give; it means identifying what the other person needs and then helping them with that.

To find out what that is, first you need to take interest in the other person. After identifying what he or she needs, decide what you will share. It doesn't necessarily have to be material. An expression of your interest and affection or time spent together could be a more delightful gift.

Name	Needs of the Person	Ways I Can Share and Help

After you've acted on your plan for sharing, close your eyes and try to get a sense for the feeling in your heart. Experience the pure joy of the soul. Write down what you feel.

_____

_____

_____

_____

_____

Sharing with Neighbors/Community

Referring to the various forms of sharing described earlier, think of what you can share and want to share with your neighbors or community in the near future. Write down your detailed plan.

Target of Sharing	Things You Can and Want to Share	Detailed Sharing/ Activity Plan	When

Act on one thing in your plan for sharing, and then write down what you felt. Close your eyes and try to sense the feeling in your heart. Experience the pure joy of the soul.

_____

_____

_____

_____

You can retire from your job, but you can't retire from life—not until you die. Your life doesn't end just because you've retired from your job. Life is the precious time and the physical power, heart power, and brain power you've been given. Whether it came from the God who created this world or the Source of the great life of the cosmos, the right to use that life energy was transferred to you the moment you were born. That right was given only to you, until you die. You're the only one who can decide how to use it. Your life energy doesn't want to be wasted meaninglessly. It wants to be used for meaningful things, for making people and the world healthier, happier, and more peaceful.

Will you put your life energy to good use as its true master, or will you be a spectator, standing by and watching with your arms folded? How would you like to do it?

_____

_____

_____

_____

What could be more satisfying than using the precious time and energy called "life" to somehow contribute to other people and the world before you die? If you let the time go by meaninglessly, won't you regret it before you died? You would likely think, "I failed to make good use of the energy of love inside me."

For what would you like to use your remaining life energy?

_____

_____

_____

_____

Enlightenment is no big deal. It's just a matter of knowing
what you really need and what others really need.
—ILCHI LEE

BE CLOSE TO NATURE

Read Chapter 12 of *I've Decided to Live 120 Years* before starting this chapter.

Nature is full of genius, full of divinity;
so that not a snowflake escapes its fashioning hand.
—HENRY DAVID THOREAU

Humans come from nature and return to nature. The embrace of nature is the ultimate refuge to which we must return. This is also the reason we should live more nature-friendly lives as we grow older. We're preparing to return from whence we came.

The benefits we receive from nature are not only the material things we use for food, clothing, and shelter. Spiritually, as well, nature can give us great wisdom and unspoken teachings. Living close to nature may provide us with all the answers to life that we've been trying so hard to find.

Letting Go of Ego in Nature

One of the fundamental causes of the suffering humans feel is the perception that "I am separate from everything else." What perceives the self as distinct from others and from the external environment is called "ego." Because our bodies are isolated from each other and we each live in our own conscious world, it's natural for us to feel separate from each other. So the ego itself is not necessarily a bad thing. The problem is the selfishness, greed, and suffering that are derived from such an awareness of separation. To escape from it, we have to move toward a consciousness that transcends the ego.

What kind of worldview do you have? Do you think that everyone is separate from one another, or do you think that we are all interconnected? Even if you think that we are interconnected, do you have difficulty actually applying that in your life? Write down your general idea about this issue.

Let's go out into nature now and meditate. You don't necessarily have to go far. A yard outside your home, a nearby park, or a walking trail will work fine.

Sit in a secluded place and look around you. Think of yourself, the subject, looking at nature, the object. Can you feel the beauty and peacefulness of nature? You're now viewing and appreciating nature. What does nature look like? Write down what you're feeling.

Now try switching your perspective. Imagine that it's not you looking at nature, but nature looking at you. Nature is the subject, and you are the object. Think of yourself as a guest visiting the place where sky, ground, rocks, and trees have always been. Understand that the nature surrounding you—the ground and sky—is the original master, and that you are a guest who has stopped by for a moment and will soon be on your way. Try to feel what nature is saying to you when you view yourself from its perspective. After taking plenty of time to meditate, write down what you felt.

Now let's approach this on a new level. Eliminate the subject-object distinction between you and nature. See yourself included as part of the nature that surrounds you. You do not exist apart from nature; you're just part of it. You are nature itself, one of many organisms in nature. Listen to what nature is saying to you. After taking plenty of time to meditate, write down what you felt.

Right now, in this very moment, when you feel that you're one with nature, has the power of your ego—which once considered you separate from all things—been strengthened or weakened?

_____

_____

_____

_____

_____

There is a really big difference between knowing as just a thought or piece of information and actually feeling and experiencing that "I am one with nature." Were you able to experience the difference? If you were, what realization did that experience bring to you?

_____

_____

_____

_____

_____

All of us in this world are a part of nature. We are a part of the global ecosystem that is interconnected by the same bioenergy field in the same space, the planet Earth. Realize that you and others—you and other organisms—are not separate from each other, that we are all one. The breath of nature enters your nostrils, granting you vitality, and the food of nature enters your mouth, creating your body. Sooner or later your body, too, will scatter and be returned to nature. When you realize that you are a natural phenomenon cycling through this massive circle of life, the ego that once separated you from all things will easily tuck tail and run.

Letting go of the ego isn't made possible by some kind of deep philosophical thinking or profound knowledge. If you just go out into nature and really open your heart, you will be assimilated by the energy of nature. Becoming nature, our original form—that is the easiest way to let go of ego. We become most natural when we are in nature.

Befriending Nature

We need friends with whom we can share our hearts. If you can open your heart and have a frank conversation with someone—whether it's a family member, a lover, a friend, a colleague, or a neighbor—that person is your precious friend.

If you have even one true friend you can share your heart with, rely on, and get help from when things are hard, then you can say that you have been very lucky.

What kind of friends do you have? Write down the friend you're closest to.

Name: _____

Relationship: _____

How did you meet that friend, and how have you helped and influenced each other as you've maintained your relationship?

_____

_____

_____

_____

_____

_____

Have you had difficulties in your close personal relationships? Have you ever felt disappointment in your personal relationships because, for example, the other person didn't satisfy you as much as you had hoped, he or she expected too much from you, or you discovered incompatibilities between the two of you? Write down any such experiences.

Have you ever avoided personal relationships, thinking that you'd be better off alone than rubbing up against other people? Have you ever felt lonely because you needed but couldn't find a friend who really understood you? Write down any such experiences.

Times when we conflict with the people we're closest to are really hard. If you fully open your heart to another person but then they betray your hopes, the resulting hurt and sense of betrayal will scar you. You will soon close your heart, because you don't want to be hurt anymore.

With nature, though, we don't need to worry about those clashes. Why? Because nature doesn't judge us. She accepts and embraces us just as we are. She's a warm refuge we can rely on for rest when things get tough, an affectionate friend who encourages us and tells us to have hope and courage.

Spend time with a good friend, nature. Go outside and commune with nature. But there is something you should keep in mind if you sincerely want to know that friend. You have to open your heart.

What do you think it means to "open your heart"? How do you open your heart? Write down your thoughts in light of your experiences with friends in the past.

_____

_____

_____

_____

_____

I think that opening your heart means becoming honest. It means frankly laying out your worries and problems, as well as your present condition and feelings. "I'm having a hard time because of such and such. These are the things I'm worried about. What should I do? Please comfort me." Unburden yourself to nature, sharing all your worries and problems. Nature will completely accept you and comfort you just as you are, and it may give you definite messages of wisdom that could resolve your concerns.

Ways to Commune with Nature

Use these different ways to connect with nature, shed your worries, and feel your own true nature as often as you can.

- Charge up with warm energy in the sunshine.
- Receive fresh life energy and learn patience while watching the trees.
- Feel the mystery and beauty of life while looking at flowers.
- Expand your mind while lying on the grass and looking up into the sky.
- Listen to the sound of water and let your worries and stress flow away from you.
- Receive the majestic, brilliant power of the sun while watching the sunrise.
- Take to heart the beauty and all the colors of the sunset.
- Feel your divinity in the cosmos while looking up into the night sky and watching the stars.

You can use the guided meditation CDs *Nature Heals* and *Nature Awakens*, which I created as resources for the nature meditations listed above. To find these resources, visit BestLifeMedia.com.

Try one of these methods today or within a few days. What nature friend will you meet, when and where? Write down your plan.

Commune with nature as you planned. Really open your heart and share your worries and problems with nature. Receive comfort and messages from nature. Then write down the conversation and feelings you shared with nature as you did these nature meditations, describing what they were like and what you felt.

Try writing a short poem about the things you felt today, like the poem on page 255 of *I've Decided to Live 120 Years*. Describe the thrill of befriending nature and the inspiration you received through that friend.

To draw closer to nature in your daily life, use the environment near your home. Search for and write down the details of a mountain, park, or other location in your vicinity that you can visit often for a more nature-friendly life. It's also good to go somewhere new, a place you've never been before.

Being Charged with Nature's Complete Energy

We are organisms made up of energy. We need energy for our souls as well as energy for our bodies. People thirst for spiritual energy that can enrich their souls and give them new inspiration.

In your life, how are you charging yourself with spiritual energy for enriching your soul? Describe this by dividing it into categories: personal relationships and the sense of achievement attained through daily/social activities, hobbies, and spiritual pursuits. Indicate a satisfaction score for each of these, and write down your reason for your low/high level of satisfaction.

Personal Relationships

Through what personal relationships are you charging your spiritual energy, and how?

Your soul's level of satisfaction?   (   ) %

What is the reason for your low/ high level of satisfaction?

Daily/Social Activities

Through what daily/social activities are you charging your spiritual energy, and how?

Your soul's level of satisfaction?   (   ) %

What is the reason for your low/ high level of satisfaction?

Hobbies

Through what hobbies are you charging your spiritual energy, and how?

Your soul's level of satisfaction? (   )%

What is the reason for your low/ high level of satisfaction?

Spiritual Pursuits

Through what spiritual pursuits are you charging your spiritual energy, and how?

Your soul's level of satisfaction? (   ) %

What is the reason for your low/ high level of satisfaction?

We pursue completeness or wholeness. Our lives are spent wandering in search of wholeness, of something that can satisfy us completely. It's not easy, though, to feel complete satisfaction in life. When we feel an emptiness, as if our souls are unfulfilled, how should we fill that space?

We can become charged with complete energy in nature. Nature is giving us the energy of infinite love and blessings—and it doesn't even tell us to give it the glory or demand anything in return. Energy containing unconditional love and blessings, that is the reason nature fulfills our souls.

Take time to recharge with the life energy of nature. Go outside on a sunny day and sit or lie down for just a moment, letting everything go in the embrace of nature. Enjoy your fill of the warm sunshine and clean air, of the fresh smell of grass and earth, of a gentle breeze, of nature's infinite energy of love.

Just accept the energy that nature gives without thinking at all. There are no conditions here. Nothing at all will be asked of you in return. Just accept it, without concern.

Take time to charge yourself with the full energy of nature. Then describe what you did, where, and what you felt.

_____

_____

_____

_____

_____

You have other parents in addition to your physical parents. These are your cosmic parents. The energy of heaven and earth caused you to be born in this land; it fed you and raised you. Try to feel that you have great cosmic parents and give yourself to their embrace, enjoying your fill of their love. And try to hear the messages your cosmic parents are giving you. Look at yourself as the mind of heaven and the mind of earth. If your cosmic parents were to see you, how would they feel, and how would they want you to live? What would they say to you? Write down what you felt through this meditation.

_____

_____

_____

_____

Growing to Be Like Nature

At your side is a great teacher, one who will fill you with inspiration and teach you wisdom in life. This teacher is nature. Students are bound to resemble their teachers. In the same way, the closer we grow to nature, the more we take on its characteristics.

What character traits did you discover in nature through your communion with it? Write down your feelings in the following spaces. If there is some area for which you can't yet get a specific feeling, first do nature meditation and then write down your feelings.

Example: Sunshine is **bright** and **warm**.
I felt **unconditional love and warmth** through sunshine.
I want to take on the **(loving) character** of sunshine.

- **Sunshine**

  Sunshine is _____ .

  I felt _____ through sunshine.

  I want to take on the (_____) character of sunshine.

- **The skies**

  The skies are _____ .

  I felt _____ through the skies.

  I want to take on the (_____) character of the skies.

- **The earth**

  The earth is _____ .

  I felt _____ through the earth.

  I want to take on the (_____) character of the earth.

- **Trees**

  Trees are _____ .

  I felt _____ through trees.

  I want to take on the (_____) character of trees.

- **Sunset**

  The sunset is _____ .

  I felt _____ through the sunset.

  I want to take on the (_____) character of the sunset.

- **Birds**

  Birds are _____ .

  I felt _____ through birds.

  I want to take on the (_____) character of birds.

Write down other characteristics that you want to develop through communion with nature—with the ocean, mountains, rivers, rocks, flowers, the sunrise, the moon, and the stars, for instance.

_____

_____

_____

_____

_____

From among the character traits you wrote before, choose the one you feel that you need most right now. Set up a plan to put it into practice in your life this week.

- Character Trait I Need Most Now: _____

- Action Plan:

_____

_____

_____

After putting this into practice in your life for a week, write down what you did and what you felt.

_____

_____

_____

_____

I encourage you to try setting up and acting on a plan for all the character traits you want to develop through nature, using a method like the one above.

Life isn't that difficult or complicated when you look at it a certain way. That's the way nature is, and that's the way you are, too. You only have to feel and act on what your teacher, nature, teaches you. That is the life of a natural person, one who grows to resemble nature.

Our deaths aren't that difficult or complicated, either. We've come from nature, and all we have to do is to live lives that resemble nature, until the time we go back to nature. The embrace of nature is ultimately the place to which we return. Let's not fear death or feel that it is strange. We're going back to where we were in the first place. It's only natural that everything in the world changes. Death appears to be the end when viewed in terms of physical life, but it is merely an event through which our life energy changes into another form.

In this world, everything seems to have a beginning and an end. But viewed from the world of energy, everything merely changes and circulates according to the eternal cosmic law of energy, without beginning and without end.

Read a portion of the *Chun Bu Kyung*, an ancient Korean text that expresses this enlightenment clearly in 81 characters, and meditate on its meaning.

一始無始 *(Il Shi Mu Shi)*
一析三極無盡本 *(Il Suk Sahm Geuk Mu Jin Bon)*
妙衍萬往萬來 *(Myo Yun Mahn Wang Mahn Rae)*
用變不動本 *(Yong Byun Bu Dong Bon)*
本心本太陽昂明 *(Bon Shim Bon Tae Yang Ang Myung)*
人中天地一 *(In Joong Chun Ji Il)*
一終無終一 *(Il Jong Mu Jong Il)*

Everything begins in one, but that one has no beginning.

One is divided into three, but its source is not expended.

Of the three, heaven is the one that emerged first, earth is the one that emerged second, and humanity is the one that emerged third.

All things mysteriously come and go within the order of the cosmos, and, although their purposes change, their Source does not change.

*Our original mind is like the sun and seeks brightness;
heaven and earth exist within humanity as one.*

Everything ends in one, but that one is without ending.

How were you inspired through this *Chun Bu Kyung* passage?

_____

_____

_____

_____

_____

_____

Do you want to live the life of a person who increasingly takes on the characteristics of nature? What does this kind of life look like to you, and what kind of death do you want to meet by living this way?

_____

_____

_____

_____

_____

_____

_____

_____

Read the poem by Nancy Wood on page 260 of *I've Decided to Live 120 Years*. Now try to picture the moment of the death you hope for. Imagine and describe in detail when, in what environment, with what expression on your face, and in what state of mind you will meet death. If you can, express what you visualize as a poem.

Everything begins in One and ends in One, but that One is eternal without beginning or end. Awakening to the One and returning to it is Chunhwa.

—ILCHI LEE

WHAT WE LEAVE BEHIND

Read Chapter 13 of *I've Decided to Live 120 Years* before starting this chapter.

> *Never doubt that a small group of thoughtful, committed citizens*
> *can change the world; indeed, it's the only thing that ever has.*
> —MARGARET MEAD

Planning a Lifestyle for Your Old Age

The rapid increase in the older population is advance notice that the social influence of the elderly is expanding, and this phenomenon is already conspicuous in several long-lived countries. Will the growth in the older population act as a force for upgrading society or as a burden on the next generation? This is an issue that will determine our future.

Although different forms of institutional support from society will, of course, be needed, the answer to that question depends more fundamentally on the awareness of the elderly and on what lifestyles they choose. We again need to see older people serving as mentors for younger people, which was the norm in traditional society long ago. For that to happen, the consciousness of the elderly must awaken.

Think about your childhood. Do you have a memory of communicating with an older person among your immediate family, other relatives, or neighbors? Write down how that person treated and influenced you and the people around you.

_____

_____

_____

_____

_____

What thoughts come to mind when you see older people these days? What do you feel when you see a wise, kind senior? When you see a stubborn, self-centered senior?

_____

_____

_____

_____

_____

Do you believe that the way of life you personally choose can affect the people around you? Write down any experience you've had with your lifestyle affecting those around you, or with the lifestyles of others affecting you.

In your old age, how do you want to appear to the people around you and to the next generation? Picture, and then write down in detail, the image, attitude, way of life, and activities that comprise this picture.

▶ Image of Old Age:

▶ Attitude:

_____

_____

_____

_____

▶ Way of Life:

_____

_____

_____

_____

▶ Activities:

_____

_____

_____

_____

Living as an Earth Citizen

Global climate change and environmental pollution are not threats to the distant future; they are with us now. We humans did this; no one else is to blame. At a basic level, our lives are already being shaken by water we can't drink without worrying, air we can't breathe with peace of mind, food we can't eat without concern over chemicals and genetic manipulation, and massive patches of plastic garbage contaminating our oceans and seafood.

Bring to mind the environment as it was when you were young. Now try to feel how much worse environmental pollution has become compared with that time. You'll feel it immediately if you just think of water, air, and food. Write down the discomfort and anxiety you feel in your daily life due to climate change and environmental pollution.

What attitude do you have toward global environmental problems? Are you thinking in a passive way, "Somebody will take care of it; leaders and experts will know what to do"? Are you thinking of it pessimistically, "The world won't change no matter what anybody does"? Or are you acting even in little things with the attitude that your small actions are the beginning of great change? Reflect on and describe your personal attitude.

Can you believe that 40 percent of the global death rate is due to environmental pollution and that 1.7 million children per year are dying from the same cause? Environmental pollution is threatening human life. What do you think is the fundamental cause of environmental pollution?

American environmental activist Gus Speth said, "I used to think that top environmental problems were biodiversity loss, ecosystem collapse, and climate change. I thought that 30 years of good science could address these problems. I was wrong. The top environmental problems are selfishness, greed, and apathy, and to deal with these we need a cultural and spiritual transformation. And we scientists don't know how to do that."

Do you sympathize with Dr. Speth? Why do you think people cause environmental issues out of selfishness, greed, and disinterest?

Disinterest in the global environment begins in a lack of awareness that "the earth is my home." Earth Citizens are people who think of the earth as their home and other people as family members who share that home. The first step for a good Earth Citizen's life is to have hope and ownership of your life. Those who have no sense of ownership or who have lost hope for their own lives will have the same kind of thinking about the planet.

Do you have a sense of ownership and hope for your own life? Do you agree that the ownership and responsibility you feel for your life are directly connected with your attitude toward the environment of the planet?

_____

_____

_____

_____

_____

I believe that everyone hopes for the health and happiness of all other people and lives, as well as their own, and that they have a desire to contribute, even if only a little, to making the world a better place. I believe that you, too, definitely have that hope and desire. Try to sense what you truly feel and express those feelings in writing.

_____

_____

_____

_____

_____

_____

Read the story of Hanabuchi Keiko, introduced on pages 276 to 279 of *I've Decided to Live 120 Years*, and then write down what you felt while reading it.

Do you want to burn with passion for some precious value until the last moment of your life, like Hanabuchi Keiko? If you do, write down how you want to express and realize that desire.

If you have that desire, that is the mind of an Earth Citizen. And acting on it is the life of an Earth Citizen. If you're curious about the Earth Citizens Movement or want to take part in it, I hope you will go to www.EarthCitizens.org, watch the video on earth citizenship, and register as an Earth Citizen.

The following is a list of documentaries containing messages about the seriousness of global environmental pollution and climate change. The subjects of these films (available as videos) are shown in parentheses. I hope that you will watch these one by one, beginning with the areas of particular interest to you, and that, as a member of the global community living in these times, you will continue to expand the shared consensus on these important issues.

- *Last Call at the Oasis* (Participant Media, 2011, water crisis)
- *A Crude Awakening: The Oil Crash* (Lava Productions, 2016, oil/energy)
- *Wasted! The Story of Food Waste* (Zero Point Zero Production, 2017)
- *Food, Inc.* (Magnolia Pictures et al., 2008, unhealthy food industry)
- *Racing Extinction* (Oceanic Preservation Society et al., 2015, biodiversity)
- *This Changes Everything* (Klein Lewis Productions et al., 2015, climate)
- *An Inconvenient Truth* (Lawrence Bender Productions, 2006, climate)
- *An Inconvenient Sequel: Truth to Power* (Actual Films et al., 2017, energy)

I believe seniors have a responsibility to show that the completion of their personal lives contributes to making a more humane and mature society, and I believe they have the potential and power to do that. Deciding to live to be 120 doesn't mean that you merely want to live a long time; it's an expression of your conviction and will to change your life, change your community, and set the human species and the earth on course to a better future.

I believe in the power of the dreams that people have. The great dream of one person could stop with changing his or her life, but a great dream embraced by many people could change the world. A desire for other people and life forms, as well as themselves, to be healthy and happy and to contribute to creating a better world, that is the great human spirit, the dream and truth quickening in all our hearts.

Through that dream, we will finally be connected as one!

Do you believe in the power of dreams? Do you have that great heart, that great dream within you, too? If you do, then show that heart and realize that dream. What will you choose to make the dream come true?

What today's senior generation, the longest-lived generation in the history of our species, can leave on the earth will be determined by what values each person pursues and how each of us lives. A way of life for experiencing true inner joy and maturity of character through sharing, giving, and heading toward completion—that is a way of life that will create a new culture of aging and act as a true and powerful force for changing the world.

Like the crimson leaves of autumn burning with passion for their final moment, like a sunset ending the day with the most brilliant, majestic colors, let us make the twilight of our lives glow brilliantly. Though our bodies decline and weaken, the essence of our spirits will grow in splendor and magnificence.

The world is not a collection of separate things;
everything is interconnected by energy.
—ILCHI LEE

FEEL YOURSELF AND ALL PEOPLE, HERE AND NOW

Congratulations on finishing all chapters of this workbook. I'm guessing that you have traveled far and wide in your journey as you reflected on 13 different topics. You went into your past, into the life you have lived up until now. You went deep inside yourself to look at your thoughts, emotions, and soul. Through a journey into your brain, you gave it messages of hope, and you also journeyed into the self-image you dream of and into your future and old age.

I want to applaud your courage. It probably wasn't all that easy to take an honest look at who you really are. You do this only if you have an honest courage that seeks to face your truth, not external packaging or falsehood. We gain a level of maturity, become more magnanimous, and gradually learn the principles of life by having the courage to see the truth of ourselves just as we are. Was that true for you on your journey?

You've finished your excursion into these 13 areas, but I hope you'll take the time to reflect on that process again. You'll be able to discover a still deeper level of meaning when you take this journey a step further and gain additional lessons from it. Ask yourself the following questions.

As you went on this journey, how honest were you with yourself? How much did you try to see yourself just as you are? Are you satisfied with your efforts?

How did you grow and change through this journey? Look back at your answers on page 78. What internal, external, or lifestyle changes have you experienced in the process of completing this workbook? Write them down, comparing yourself now with who you were before setting out on your journey.

▶ Before:

▶ After:

What part of this journey impressed you most deeply, and why? What was your greatest realization? Did you experience some positive change in your thinking or life as a result?

What part of this journey was the hardest for you? Did you have difficulty facing and acknowledging some part of who you really are? When was that, and why was it difficult? How did you overcome this, and what did you learn as a result?

Through this journey, what have you come to understand and accept more fully about yourself?

Through this journey, what have you come to understand and tolerate more fully about the people around you?

Through this journey, what have you come to understand and embrace more fully about life and about the world?

Summarize and organize your design for your future by considering the following questions.

What is the central value you want to pursue through your life in the future?

How many years have you decided to live?

Why did you choose that age?

Write in detail what you want to achieve with the lifespan you've chosen.

_____

_____

_____

_____

What virtues will you focus on cultivating during that time?

_____

_____

_____

_____

Summarize your detailed plan for the three areas of a spiritual, completion-directed life:

1. Life of Spiritual Practice:

_____

_____

_____

2. Life of Sharing (Hongik):

_____

_____

_____

3. Life of a Natural Person:

_____

_____

_____

Remember the mission statement you wrote on page 57 in Chapter 2, and look at whether there is something in it that should be revised. Write your mission statement again.

My Mission Statement:

Finally, there is something I would like to ask you to do.

Your design for the future isn't a fixed, final version. Continue to update it as you go forward. Develop it in a direction that is more detailed and more positive, in a direction that benefits yourself, the people around you, and the world. Then your energy field will expand and connect to more people and to the world.

The future is always open. What you choose now, in this moment, may affect an hour or a day of your time, or it may affect your whole life. Your future is awaiting you with boundless possibilities. Become the master of that time and space.

Feel yourself and all people, here and now. Awaken to the self that is breathing in this space and time, to the self that is interconnected with all things. That realization is the light of your awakened soul.

And create. Express your life and actualize the reason for your existence through creation. Let the light of life move and shine. And enjoy your fill of joy and peace within that light.

Remember that you, like light, are a being of brightness, warmth, and wisdom. You have a wholeness that cannot be compared with anyone else. Bring out that wholeness. Actualize it. The completion-directed life will lead you.

NOTES

ACKNOWLEDGMENTS

I'd like to extend my gratitude to the many people who helped in the creation of this workbook or gave it their support. I couldn't have done it without them.

From beginning to end, Hyerin Moon, Jiyoung Oh, and Michela Mangiaracina at Best Life Media put in their editing and production expertise. Daniel Graham translated the Korean manuscript into English, and Phyllis Elving turned the English into engaging and fluid text. Sue Vander Hook polished the manuscript with her proofreading skills.

The visual content contributed greatly to the effectiveness and usability of this workbook, and for that I have to thank Kiryl Lysenka for his interior and cover design, Jooyoung Ryu for her warm illustrations, and Dylan Miller for his help with the graphs.

I'd like to give special thanks to Dr. Deborah Coady and Nicole Dean, who provided valuable feedback that guided the final editing process.

ABOUT THE AUTHOR

Ilchi Lee is an impassioned visionary, educator, mentor, and innovator; he has dedicated his life to teaching energy principles and researching and developing methods to nurture the full potential of the human brain.

For more than 35 years, his life's mission has been to help people harness their own creative power and personal potential. For this goal, he has developed many successful mind-body training methods, including Body & Brain Yoga and Brain Education. His principles and methods have inspired many people around the world to live healthier and happier lives.

Lee is a *New York Times* bestselling author who has penned more than 40 books, including *The Call of Sedona: Journey of the Heart*, *Change: Realizing Your Greatest Potential*, and *The Power Brain: Five Steps to Upgrading Your Brain Operating System*.

He is also a well-respected humanitarian who has been working with the United Nations and other organizations for global peace. He began the Earth Citizen Movement, a global drive to raise awareness of the values of earth citizenship and put them into practice.

Lee serves as president of the University of Brain Education, the Global Cyber University, and the International Brain Education Association. For more information about Ilchi Lee and his work, visit Ilchi.com.

RESOURCES

Body & Brain Yoga and Tai Chi Classes

The 100 Body & Brain Yoga and Tai Chi centers in the United States are one of the best ways you can make the exercises and principles introduced in this book a meaningful part of your daily life. They offer classes, workshops, and individual sessions based on East Asian healing and energy philosophies. The expert instructors and center community also provide advice and support for your continued growth and life creation. Find a center at **BodynBrain.com**.

Retreats and Workshops

Opportunities to immerse yourself in the feeling of being one with nature, reflect on your life, and plan for its second half are offered at each of these retreat centers.

Sedona Mago Retreat

Nestled among the red rocks on a stunning 175-acre stretch of land under the wide blue sky of the high Arizona desert, Sedona Mago Retreat is an ideal place for letting nature sweep aside the hustle and bustle of a busy life. Here you will have a chance to look within to find the answers to who you are and what you really want. Go for a personal retreat to plan the second half of your life or join one of the many programs for ongoing self-development offered there. Learn more at **SedonaMagoRetreat.org**.

Honor's Haven

For a personal getaway among the rolling hills of the Shawangunk Mountain Region, the gateway to the Catskills in New York, visit Honor's Haven Resort & Spa. The 200 acres of lush gardens, crystalline lake, and meditative forest will inspire you to discover the greater you within. Enjoy wellness classes and retreat programs in which experienced instructors will guide you on your inner journey. Learn more at **HonorsHaven.com**.

I've Decided to Live 120 Years Personal Workbook Resources

Throughout this workbook, various books, videos, audio meditations, and other resources were mentioned to help you plan for a long, happy, and fulfilling life. You can find these resources or links to them gathered at **Live120YearsBook.com/resources**.

Live 120 Years Special Online Course

I've Decided to Live 120 Years springs to life in this online course. Its meditation and writing exercises walk you through the key ideas and practices featured in the book. It includes exclusive interviews with Ilchi Lee and other experts. Readers receive a special discount for the course. For more information, visit **Live120YearsCourse.com**.

One-Minute Exercise App

Author Ilchi Lee had an app developed to help you adopt One-Minute Exercise as a daily habit. Available for both iOS and Android, it includes an alarm, timer, tracker, and library of One-Minute Exercise videos to follow. You can learn more about the One Minute Change app and download it for free at **1MinuteChange.com**.

Living as an Earth Citizen begins with each individual's choice, but when many individuals come together, systemic change can begin. The Earth Citizen Movement raises awareness of the power of personal choice, promotes the spirit of earth citizenship, and spearheads real action for a healthier and sustainable world. It is coordinated by the Earth Citizens Organization (ECO), a nonprofit that trains Earth Citizen leaders and introduces ways to live mindfully and sustainably. You can learn more about an Earth Citizen lifestyle, find volunteer opportunities, join an Earth Citizen Club, and see ECO training programs at **EarthCitizens.org**.

Products of Related Interest

The following products have useful information and practices for designing your life's period of completion. See them and more of Ilchi Lee's work at **BestLifeMedia.com**.

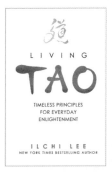

Living Tao

Timeless Principles for Everyday Enlightenment

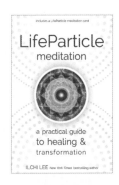

LifeParticle Meditation

A Practical Guide to Healing and Transformation

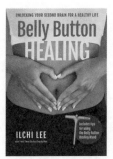

Belly Button Healing

Unlocking Your Second Brain for a Healthy Life

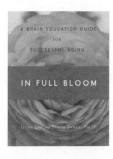

In Full Bloom

A Brain Education Guide for Successful Aging

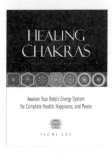

Healing Chakras

Awaken Your Body's Energy System for Complete Health, Happiness, and Peace

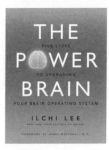

The Power Brain

Five Steps to Upgrading Your Brain Operating System

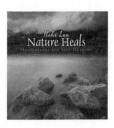

Nature Heals

Meditations for Self-Healing

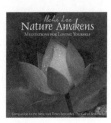

Nature Awakens

Meditations for Loving Yourself